About the Author

Larry Neild is one of the most experienced and respected tranquilliser lay workers in the country. He is co-ordinator and co-founder of Tranxline, an organisation established in Liverpool in 1983 to give advice and information to people wanting to withdraw from tranquillisers and sleeping pills. Because of his expertise he has appeared on many national television and radio programmes. He is also a professional writer specialising in health topics, particularly the promotion of natural health.

CAUTION

Under no circumstances must prescribed medication such as tranquillisers or sleeping pills be stopped abruptly. It is dangerous and will make you ill. Please read all of this book before embarking on any tablet withdrawal plan and always consult your doctor.

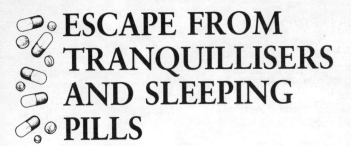

ESCAPE FROM TRANQUILLISERS AND SLEEPING PILLS

A Proven DIY Withdrawal Plan

Larry Neild

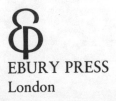

EBURY PRESS
London

First published by Ebury Press
an imprint of the Random Century Group Ltd
Random Century House
20 Vauxhall Bridge Road
London SW1V 2SA

British Library Cataloguing in Publication Data
Neild, Larry
    Escape from tranquillisers and sleeping pills.
    1. Prescription drug addiction. Self-treatment
    I. Title
    616.86068

    ISBN 0-85223-913-0

Typeset in Sabon by Tek Art Ltd, Croydon, Surrey
Printed and bound in Great Britain by
Richard Clay Limited, Bungay, Suffolk

Acknowledgements

I would to like to acknowledge the pioneering work of Joan Jerome, Anita Gordon, Ann Pitman and last, but by no means least, Shirley Trickett. I much value the friendship, support and encouragement of all of them over the years. In my own area of Merseyside I owe a special thanks to Peggy Ashton, Mary Cave and Mavis Cox for all their work and support, and to the late county councillor Tom Talbot without whose help our organisation would never have been founded. A special thanks to Dr Heather Ashton of Newcastle University for teaching me so much about this problem and for promptly answering the most difficult questions over the years, and to Ron Lacey for his campaigning work at national level.

At Ebury Press I have valued the help, support and encouragement of Rowena Webb who gently knocked me and my manuscript into shape and would like to thank, too, my copy-editor Esther Jagger for using a pen like a magic wand as she cast her literary eye over my work.

My biggest thanks goes to the thousands of people who have shared with me their laughs, cries, fears and tears over many years. None of them deserved to suffer and it is with honour and humility that I dedicate my book to them, the innocent victims.

Contents

Preface by C H Ashton, DM, FRCP and Ron Lacey

Introduction

Part I: The Problem

1   What Are Tranquillisers and How Do They Work?   17
2   What Bottled Happiness Has Done for Society   28
3   Is Escape from Tablets Possible?   52

Part II: The Escape Plan

4   The Withdrawal Diet   63
5   The Breathing Exercise   81
6   Tablet Withdrawal – Essential Ground Rules   90
7   Coming off Diazepam (Valium)   101
8   Coming off Lorazepam (Ativan)   111
9   Coming off Sleeping Pills and Other Benzodiazepines   120
10   Coming off Barbiturates and Non-Benzodiazepines   126
11   Life after Pills   134

Appendix: List of Benzodiazepines   146
Further Reading   151
Useful Addresses   153
Index   155

Preface

This book is written largely for the million or more men and women in Britain who are long-term users of benzodiazepine sleeping pills and tranquillisers. These are people who have taken the drugs in good faith, often for twenty years or more, in 'therapeutic' doses as prescribed by their doctors, in the belief that the drugs could be taken for life without ill effects. It is now clear that benzodiazepines are not so harmless as first supposed. Many who have taken them will testify that the initial effects tend to wane over time, to be replaced insidiously with a range of symptoms such as increasing anxiety, depression, blunting of emotional reactions and impairment of memory and clear-thinking. At the same time a state of dependence develops, making it difficult to stop taking the drugs.

There is now a groundswell of opinion, emanating mainly from the consumers of benzodiazepines, that when taken chronically these drugs create more problems than they solve. Consequently, many long-term users now wish to withdraw from benzodiazepines. Unfortunately, they do not always find it easy to obtain clear advice from their doctors on how to proceed with this undertaking. Many doctors are themselves bewildered and inexperienced in benzodiazepine withdrawal, and are unable to offer the confident reassurance and support needed by their equally bewildered patients.

The value of this book is that it offers a clear and concise programme of benzodiazepine withdrawal which has been tried, tested and proved to be successful for many users. It presents a positive approach with practical steps which can be followed with confidence by members of the public. It gives simple, straightfoward information about benzodiazepines and about general health, which will be useful to many who find such information difficult to obtain. Self-help and support organisations such as Tranxline have accumulated more experience of benzodiazepines than most doctors and have clearly fulfilled a public need. For this reason, the book will also be of value to doctors, whose personal experience may be limited to a few patients, compared with the hundreds who have been guided through benzodiazepine withdrawal by the author.

Although this book offers a withdrawal plan, it is important to note that withdrawal may not be a realistic or appropriate goal for everyone. Withdrawal is for those who actively wish to withdraw; it is not obligatory for long-term users who are satisfied with their health (although some may profit from further information about benzodiazepines). It is to be hoped that the current 'bad press' which the benzodiazepines are receiving will not encourage doctors to insist upon withdrawal in every case. No one should be pressurised to withdraw; the drugs should never be stopped abruptly; patients should never be threatened with a deadline. Unfortunately all these circumstances have occasionally occurred.

C H Ashton, DM, FRCP
Lecturer in Clinical Psychopharmacology
and Honorary Consultant Clinical Pharmacologist,
Newcastle upon Tyne

Today in Britain there are probably ten times more people addicted to drugs prescribed by their doctors than are addicted to illegal drugs such as heroin and cocaine. That this fact is now widely known is due to vigorous campaigning by lay people and organisations rather than to the awareness or concern of doctors or health service professionals.

Tranquilliser withdrawal self-help groups have emerged as a major health lobby in Britain. In many parts of the country self-help groups are the only source of help available to people struggling to break the tranquilliser habit. These groups have developed a knowledge about tranquillisers and methods of safely withdrawing from them based on the first-hand experience of their members. The author of this book has been working for six years directly with people withdrawing from tranquillisers and is an articulate campaigner for better services for them.

Larry Neild's book will be particularly helpful to people who, by necessity or choice, are struggling to break their tranquilliser habit alone. It will also be helpful to their relatives and friends. Quite often the understanding and support of those closest to the individual is crucial to a successful withdrawal programme. Moreover it will also provide a useful source of information and inspiration to those courageous souls who decide to band together to form their own self-help group. Larry's work and this book provide eloquent testimony to the fact that a medical degree is not an essential prerequisite to finding healthier ways to deal with our problems.

Ron Lacey
Assistant Director at Mind, 1975–1990

Introduction

This book will tell you how to 'escape' safely from tranquillisers or sleeping pills without experiencing severe withdrawal effects: even if you have taken your tablets continuously for ten, twenty or even thirty years!

You may have tried before to stop your tablets and failed. So what is different about the method outlined in this book?

It will tell you why things didn't quite work out on your previous attempts and when you learn the correct way to proceed you will be amazed at how easy it can be.

Think of tranquilliser addiction like being lost in a maze. There is always a way out . . . you just need to be guided in the right direction.

When you think of drug addiction, words such as heroin, cocaine, crack and cannabis spring to mind – drugs available only on the black market. Yet the numbers of people hooked on these and other illegal substances is small compared to the millions of men and women all over the world who are dependent on legally prescribed drugs such as tranquillisers and sleeping pills. Explaining to his children why he had been arrested for possession of marijuana, ex-Beatle Paul McCartney told them: 'It's best to live without any stimulants or relaxants – but if you want my advice on what I think are the most dangerous I'll tell you that tranquillisers and stuff like that, available on prescription from doctors, are probably the worst.'

In the United Kingdom alone, more than 3 million people each year are prescribed tranquillisers or sleeping pills or both, and a recent survey reported in the *British Journal of Addiction* revealed that 1.7 million take them for far longer than the recommended period. Indeed, at least 1.2 million take their tablets continuously for over a year, and in many cases for five, ten or even thirty years. Even the pharmaceutical companies which manufacture tranquillisers and sleeping pills warn that they should be used only for short-term treatment – a few weeks, or several months at the most. So people who find themselves hooked on tranquillisers or sleeping pills are not drug abusers or misusers, but ordinary men and women from all walks of life who at some stage have embarked on a course of treatment administered by their family doctor.

It is hard to believe that such vast numbers of people could be made ill by following a prescribed treatment, and it was this disbelief that set me off on my researches in the early 1980s, with a visit to Liverpool City Library. As I leafed through the pages of academic reading material on the scientific shelves of the reference section I was shocked to discover the 'hidden' side of everyday medicines: column after column of advice, warnings and data essentially aimed at the eyes of the medical profession. That visit sparked off a deep interest in drugs, and I began by enrolling for a course on drug counselling.

All too often these harmless-looking little tablets have been seen as the great panacea of the late twentieth century. Once described as the nearest thing to bottled happiness, the pills for all ills, they were immortalised in a sixties' Rolling Stones song, 'Mother's Little Helpers'. They have been given for backache, neckache, headaches, to help people sit exams, to cope with family deaths, to be calm before a dental appointment or driving test. Carol, for instance, a married woman in her twenties, was prescribed tranquillisers because she had a violent husband (her GP never considered that he should 'treat' the husband for his behaviour!). Brenda was given them because her young baby was hyperactive and kept her awake at night; that child was a teenager when his mother eventually managed to escape from her tablets. Ray was prescribed Valium as a muscle relaxant after being injured playing football; the 'habit' he got into as a result eventually ended his sporting days.

What concerned me most was the fact that there was hardly any help available for people caught up in the tranquilliser trap – such centres as there were had in the main been established to help hard-drug users. We are brought up to respect the words of doctors – we trust them with our health, our lives; the problem caused by these tablets has been the biggest-ever health blunder, and yet it seemed that the healthcare profession had virtually turned its back on this vast army of innocent victims. Moved by their plight, in 1983 I helped to establish an organisation in Liverpool – Tranxline – to give advice, information and new hope to people hooked on their tablets.

But the work did not stop there. I and the other co-founders of Tranxline campaigned for the sufferers of what we knew was a genuine illness. We discussed the problem with the Anglican Bishop and Roman Catholic Archbishop of Liverpool, and with the then Health Minister, Edwina Currie, and other health chiefs. I also served as a member of an official working party set up by one of the National Health Service's biggest regional authorities to look into the problems posed by tranquilliser use; my call was for decent facilities so that people caught in this web could be aided in a dignified way.

Our efforts and growing expertise caught the eye of a

number of broadcasting organisations and enabled us to spread the message further. I was a consultant adviser to Central TV during the filming of a sequence on Ativan for *The Cook Report*; and after an appearance on ITV's networked magazine programme *This Morning* thousands of letters poured in from all over the country. The BBC asked me to face an official spokesman from the British Medical Association in a TV discussion on *Daytime Live*, and to be adviser for a *Brass Tacks* documentary about tranquillisers. There have also been dozens of radio shows and interviews.

But I am convinced that real help from official sources will never become available for the vast majority, simply because of the huge numbers of people involved. So what can be done about it? We can scream from our rooftops about the unfairness of that situation, or we can seek a way out.

Many of the requests for help that I receive are from doctors wanting to know how they can help get their patients off pills that created misery rather than tranquillity. I have lectured to victims, to members of the medical profession, to university students, to trade unions, to magistrates, to probation officers . . . to anybody who will listen. By 1990 over 26,000 people had written to, telephoned or spoken to me or one of the Tranxline helpers. This book has been written for the many thousands more who are still desperate for help.

It should, however, be pointed out that it is not a substitute for health treatment and having read it through, you should then refer to your doctor before embarking on the withdrawal plan.

Part I
The Problem

1
What are Tranquillisers and How Do They Work?

What exactly are tranquillisers, and for that matter, sleeping pills? Tranquillisers such as Valium and sleeping tablets like Temazepam are members of a group of medicines available only on prescription and known as benzodiazepines. There are dozens available – some brands will be familiar household names; others you may never have heard of; and generic or chemical names are used as well as brand names. On p. 146 there is a list of chemical and brand names of the most commonly prescribed tablets in Australia, Canada, New Zealand, South Africa, the UK and the USA. It is a good idea to check through it to find out whether any of your medication is a member of this family of drugs.

Benzodiazepines are known in the medical world as 'minor tranquillisers'. Some people have wrongly assumed the word 'minor' to mean mild; but these drugs are by no means mild, and the word 'minor' merely distinguishes them from a completely different range of drugs known as 'major tranquillisers', which are used in the treatment of serious mental illnesses. In this book all references to 'tranquillisers' are to benzodiazepines – in other words 'minor tranquillisers'.

What should benzodiazepines be used for?

In medicine there are three main uses for these drugs:

○ *Anxiety:* they are widely prescribed for anxiety, life problems or acute panic attacks.

Often they are used in hospitals as a pre-med before surgery, because they calm down the patient. In this context, they are doubly useful: they help the patient forget about the 'unpleasant' surgery because they have an amnesiac effect.

○ *Hypnotics:* when it was discovered that benzodiazepines had sleep-promoting properties they became popular as 'sleeping pills', so they are also officially classified in the doctors' official reference book, *The British National Formulary*, as drugs for the short-term treatment of insomnia.

○ *Relaxants:* they are often prescribed for physical conditions such as pulled muscles, because they are powerful muscle relaxants.

Benzodiazepines are sometimes also prescribed to epileptics, but that is beyond the scope of this book.

How should benzodiazepines be used?

When they are used as tranquillisers, says the *Formulary*, the course of treatment should be for the shortest possible time. Recently more detailed advice about the prescribing of benzodiazepines has come from the Committee on the Safety of Medicines (CSM), a government medical body:

○ They are intended for the short-term relief of anxiety that is severe, disabling or subjecting the individual to unacceptable distress.

○ Their use to treat short-term 'mild' anxiety is inappropriate and unsuitable.

○ They should be used to treat insomnia only when it is severe, disabling or subjecting the individual to extreme distress. (See below for further information on the use of benzodiazepines as sleeping pills).

Confirming this advice, data information sheets produced by the pharmaceutical companies which manufacture these drugs state that the effectiveness of tranquillisers in long-term use – that is, for more than four months – has not been assessed by clinical studies.

Another source of information sent fortnightly to every doctor in the UK is a factsheet known as the *Drug and Therapeutics Bulletin*. It is produced by the Consumers' Association and edited by a highly respected pharmacologist, Dr Andrew Herxheimer of the Westminster Medical School in London. A few years ago it devoted an issue to the problems of benzodiazepines, and stated that there was evidence to suggest that regular treatments for as little as four to six weeks could lead to withdrawal problems. Not long afterwards the *Bulletin* looked at the drug Lorazepam (also known as Ativan), and concluded that its use as a tranquilliser was best limited to courses of treatment of a week or two. The most recent editions of *The British National Formulary* now follow the new guidelines issued by the Committee on the Safety of Medicines and state that all tranquillisers should be prescribed for only two to four weeks. Problems have arisen because all these prescribing guidelines have largely been ignored.

Sleeping pills

A lot of people have been heard to say: 'I don't take tranquillisers – I only take mild sleeping pills'. It comes as quite a shock when they realise that their particular 'mild sleeping pill' is a powerful tranquilliser.

Indeed they are interchangeable: if Lorazepam, a common tranquilliser, is taken at bedtime it becomes a sleeping pill. Similarly – though it is not usual – Temazepam taken in the day becomes a tranquilliser. The unfortunate result is that a person can be on two or more different benzodiazepine drugs at once: no wonder the brain finds it hard to function.

Very often a person taking a tranquilliser may start to have disturbed sleep or insomnia, possibly due to a side effect. In many cases a doctor responds to this situation by prescribing sleeping pills. Doctors do, by and large, issue sleeping pills with the very best intentions, firmly believing that a patient desperate for sleep needs something to help. But the leading medical handbooks suggest that it is inappropriate for people to be on different benzodiazepine drugs at the same time.

The guidelines in the doctors' *Formulary* about the use of benzodiazepines as 'sleeping pills' list three stages of insomnia or sleep problems, and suggest how the drugs should be used in each case.

O *Transient insomnia:* caused by jet lag, noise, shift work, etc. If a sleeping pill is appropriate the doctor should prescribe just one or two tablets. But how many GPs would write out a prescription for a single tablet? And how would patients react to paying a full prescription charge for a bottle containing no more than a couple of pills?

○ *Short-term insomnia:* may last a few weeks or recur. Sleeping pills *may* be useful but should not be given for more than three weeks and preferably only one week. Intermittent use may also be helpful – in other words taking sleeping pills for one or two nights, then having a few weeks without before taking them again for one or two nights. The advantage of intermittent or occasional use is that it avoids the risks of people becoming dependent on sleeping pills. If pills must be taken it is better to have a couple of good nights' (drugged) sleep a fortnight than to take pills every night with the inherent risks.

○ *Chronic insomnia:* This, says the *Formulary*, is rarely benefited by sleeping pills. People who suffer from long-term insomnia should consult their GP to discuss alternative solutions that don't involve sleeping pills.

What are the right dosages?

All benzodiazepines have different strengths; for instance, a person taking 1mg of Lorazepam would be on a different level of drug dosage than somebody taking 1mg of Diazepam. The following list gives an indication of the normal adult therapeutic doses of the most commonly prescribed benzodiazepines. It should be remembered that elderly people would normally take half the usual adult dose. For other brand names not mentioned here see the list on p. 146.

Tranquillisers

Chemical name	Main UK brand name	Available in these forms	Normal dose
Diazepam	Valium	tablets: 2mg, 5mg and 10mg; capsules: 2mg and 5mg; suppositories: 10mg; liquids: 2mg per 5 ml (teaspoon)	2mg three times daily, increased in severe anxiety to 15–30mg daily in divided doses. For insomnia: 5–15mg at bedtime.
Alprazolam	Xanax	tablets: 250mcg and 500mcg	250–500mcg three times daily, increased if necessary to a total of 3mg daily.
Bromazepam	Lexotan	tablets: 1.5 (1½) mg and 3mg	3–18mg daily in divided doses. Maximum dose in hospital patients 60mg daily in divided doses.

Chemical name	Main UK brand name	Available in these forms	Normal dose
Chlordiazepoxide	Librium	tablets: 5mg, 10mg and 25mg; capsules: 5mg and 10mg	10mg three times daily, increased in severe anxiety to 100mg daily in divided doses.
Clobazam	Frisium	capsules: 10mg	20mg–30mg daily in divided doses or as a single dose at bedtime. In hospital patients it can be increased to a maximum of 60mg daily in divided doses.
Chlorazepate Dipotassium	Tranxene	capsules: 7.5 (7½) mg and 15mg	7.5 (7½)– 22.5 (22½) mg daily in two or three divided doses, or as a single dose of 15mg at bedtime.
Ketazolam	Anxon	capsules: 15mg and 30mg	30mg at bedtime, adjusted according to response.

Chemical name	Main UK brand name	Available in these forms	Normal dose
(Ketazolam continued)			Adult range is 15–60mg daily as a single dose at bedtime, or in divided doses.
Lorazepam	Ativan	tablets: 1mg and 2.5 (2½) mg	1–4mg daily in divided doses. For insomnia, 1–4mg at bedtime.
Medazepam	Nobrium	capsules: 5mg and 10mg	15–30mg daily in divided doses, increased in severe anxiety to a maximum of 40mg daily in divided doses.
Oxazepam	Oxanid	tablets: 10mg, 15mg and 30mg; capsules: 30mg	15–30mg three or four times daily.

Sleeping pills

Flurazepam	Dalmane	capsules: 15mg and 30mg	15–30mg 30 minutes before bedtime.

Chemical name	Main UK brand name	Available in these forms	Normal dose
Loprazolam	Dormonoct	tablets: 1mg	1mg at bedtime, increased if required to 1.5 (1½) mg or 2mg.
Lormetazepam	Lormetazepam	tablets: 500 mcg and 1mg	1mg at bedtime.
Nitrazepam	Mogadon	tablets: 5mg and 10mg; capsules: 5mg; liquids: 2.5 (2½) mg per 5 ml (teaspoon)	5–10mg 30 minutes before bedtime.
Temazepam	Normison	tablets: 10mg and 20mg; capsules: 10mg, 15mg, 20mg and 30mg; liquids: 10 mg per 5 ml (teaspoon)	10–30mg immediately before bedtime, increasing in severe insomnia to 60mg at bedtime.
Triazolam	Halcion	tablets: 125 mcg and 250 mcg	250mcg 15–30 minutes before bedtime.

How tranquillisers and sleeping pills work

In medical language, benzodiazepines interfere with chemical activity in the brain and nervous system by reducing communication between nerve cells. To put it more simply, in normal circumstances the human body produces its very own 'natural tranquillisers' and chemicals which help us cope with the stresses and strains of everyday life. They also enable us to sleep. Imagine it in terms of a reservoir. Normally there are enough natural chemicals in your own reservoir to deal with everyday life; but then something upsetting happens such as a bereavement or a divorce or moving house, and the need for stress-coping chemicals becomes greater. The body's reservoir is limited, so you top up with a synthetic chemical such as Diazepam or Lorazepam.

When a tranquilliser is swallowed it travels into the stomach, is 'processed' through the digestive system, and hitches a ride through the bloodstream into the brain. There it heads for what to all intents and purposes is the control room, from where it influences the natural processes which control calmness, wakefulness, anxiety and even the physical workings of the body. In effect tranquillisers damp down the brain, and for short-term use in an emergency this is acceptable.

The tranquilliser trap

The trouble is that when the tranquillisers are taken continuously for weeks or months the brain reaches the stage where it may not be able to work without them. This is what being 'hooked on tablets' really means – you need to take the tablets so that your brain, and hence your body, can function.

This chemical impact has a very powerful physical effect on the brain. Your body's own natural reservoir is temporarily switched off, and the job of controlling how you feel and how you cope with everyday stresses is left in the hands of the tablet or capsule. Your own brain will previously have produced its own natural tranquilliser on-tap, depending on the amount needed at any given time. Now imagine what happens when you have to rely solely on the tablets. Your brain gets a specific amount, day in, day out – sometimes too much, usually not enough. That is why it is so common for long-term users of tranquillisers to feel ill on a daily basis while taking their usual doses of tablets.

To make matters even worse, the brain becomes tolerant to a particular level of drug and starts to need more to do the same job. So to keep on top of things people need more tablets – but that just ensures that they get ensnared more deeply in the tranquilliser trap. In a few cases people have taken more than the ordinary therapeutic doses, and it is easy to understand why: their brain is screaming out for more of the drug. This does not imply weakness on their part, but a real physical need for chemical tranquillisation.

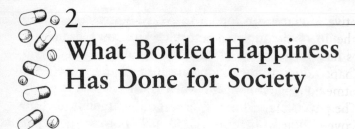

2
What Bottled Happiness
Has Done for Society

Tranquillisers and their close relatives, sleeping pills, became the biggest-ever money-spinners for the drugs industry during the sixties, seventies and eighties. They are just part of man's quest for 'medicines' to take the edge off life's stresses and strains, and that search is still continuing as scientists strive to perfect new, better and safer products. But according to Dr Heather Ashton, a highly respected psychopharmacologist from Newcastle University, we would not be any worse off if they had never been discovered. So how did we arrive at this sorry state of affairs?

A few thousand years ago Greek and Egyptian doctors dispensed them in the form of herbal medicines. The Aztecs of Central America found mushrooms with a calming effect, and in the Far East hashish was used. Over the centuries all manner of things have been done to people to 'cure' them of physical and mental illnesses. They have been dipped into water, scalded, had spirits driven out of them. But the simple act of 'swallowing' something has for thousands of years been the most common method of achieving a cure. Everything from herbs to the most dubious concoctions have been religiously 'swallowed' as medicine. Some centuries back powdered snakeroot became popular and was sold, often by travelling 'medicine men', to help cure 'mental agitation'. A modern-day relative of that remedy is still around – it was introduced in the 1950s as meprobamate. Every society through the ages had something to deal with stress and pain. Today, perhaps because of so many 'drug' disasters, herbal treatment is enjoying a revival.

The pill revolution had its origins in a remarkable little discovery two hundred years ago. Previously doctors had had to make tablets laboriously by hand, but then an artist from Devon invented a way of making them using a die or press. In due course that led to the birth of pharmaceutical companies, and soon the age of the drugs industry had arrived.

In 1869 the first synthetic drug, chloral, came on to the market; it is still available to this day. Other early drug remedies, such as bromides, introduced during the reign of Queen Victoria, have survived into the twentieth century and are likely to be around in the twenty-first.

In the 1860s research work started on what was to become one of the most popular drug types of the mid-twentieth century, the barbiturates. Their research and development lasted many decades before they exploded on to the scene in the 1930s. Today in the UK an estimated 250,000 people continue to take barbiturates every day – mainly elderly people who were first prescribed them many years ago.

But doctors recognised that there were drawbacks with the barbiturates. They were so powerful a person only needed to take a small handful for disastrous or even fatal consequences. Some people died through accidentally overdosing, while others overdosed deliberately to commit suicide.

The origins of modern tranquillisers

Just before the start of the twentieth century, work had started on two new chemicals known as benzophenones and heptoxdiazines. You have probably never heard of those two substances, yet if you look closely at their names you can see that the tranquillisers which are the focus of this book, the benzodiazepines, had already arrived, albeit in embryonic form – *benzo*phenones and heptox*diazines*. Research on the two chemicals continued for several decades, but the results were not particularly encouraging. Then new tests in the 1950s produced exciting results.

These new benzodiazepines were hypnotic, sedative and relaxed muscles. They could even control wild animals. In July 1960 journalists from Fleet Street, radio and TV, were invited to a press conference in London to be told about the first of the new wonder drugs. The *Daily Mirror* carried a front-page splash with the headline proclaiming: 'WHAT THIS NEW DRUG CAN DO TO A WILD, WILD LYNX'. In the *Daily Mail* Hugh McLeave wrote, 'Doctors in Britain are being introduced to a revolutionary new drug which can transform the most ferocious animal into a docile hand-licking pet.' He said the drug could be the biggest boon yet to doctors.

Librium capsules had arrived on the scene.

The drug was discovered after many attempts by the American branch of the Swiss firm Roche. For the previous few months Librium had been tested on animals, patients, even criminals in the state prison at Houston, Texas. Dr John Kinross-Wright, who studied the effects of Librium on the prisoners, revealed that they were men with life-long histories of antisocial behaviour. Even in the peniten-tiary they represented a major problem, mutilating themselves, starting fires and instigating fights. 'With Librium it has been possible to maintain most of them in a placid but alert state despite their tension-provoking environment,' he said at the launch of Librium. 'From these results it might be predicted that the compound would be of use in conduct disturbances in children and adolescents.'

According to the *Daily Mail*, it was unrelated to previous tranquillising drugs and so free from their side effects.

Just two days after the *Mail* article, the *News Chronicle* warned readers, 'Do not take this drug unless a doctor tells you.' Librium, the drug that would tame a fierce tiger, was now on sale for a few shillings. The new drug was still waiting to be brought under restrictions which would prohibit its supply without a prescription.

The drug quickly became a household name and within three years its makers introduced what was to become the best seller of all in the tranquilliser world, diazepam, better known to millions as Valium.

In the years that followed many other variations arrived, and even today there is a long list of benzodiazepine preparations available. As early patents expired other manufacturers started to make copies of the benzodiazepines, often giving them their own less well known brand names. Thousands have fallen into the tranquilliser trap because of this army of names which often presents no clues as to what they actually are.

As Dr Ashton has pointed out, 'patients should not be afraid to ask on receiving a prescription, such questions as, "What does it do?", "What adverse effects might it have?", "How long should I take it for?" and "What happens when I stop it?" Even if we doctors don't always know the answers, they encourage more thoughtful prescribing.'

Who takes tranquillisers and sleeping pills?

Hooked housewives, sick superstars

They have been prescribed for people from the cosmopolitan capitals of the world to remote settlements in Africa; from sedate country villages to the cities of the world that never sleep. They are taken by the rich and famous, and by legions of people living on council estates or in suburbia – they ignore class, colour, income or any other social divisions.

Superstar Liza Minnelli was prescribed Valium for tension and grief when her famous mother, Judy Garland, died in 1969. She once said in an interview: 'Nobody takes a pill to become addicted to drugs. It's the build-up in your system that finally brings you down . . . you are dealing with chemicals that are baffling, cunning and powerful.' She sought help from the Betty Ford Center in California after saying to her sister Lorna, 'I'm sick and tired of being sick and tired.' Yet another superstar went for help to the Center established by the wife of the former American President. Elizabeth Taylor said she had taken sleeping pills every night for twenty-five years.

The one thing that all these victims have in common is that the great majority are women. Modern medicine has invented stereotypes of women as emotional, sensitive, introverted, and physically and psychologically weak. Various interpretations of the beliefs of Sigmund Freud have attributed these 'deficiencies' in women to biological factors. Women have therefore been targeted as the sector of society most likely to need, or to think they need, tranquillisers. American mental health consultant Muriel Nellis has commented, 'In their search for meaningful, comfortable or healthy traditional lives women have fallen prey to the medical industry's Pandora's box of packaged promises which all too often contains punishment.'

The persuasion game

In the 1960s the pharmaceutical industry, not surprisingly, embarked on a major promotion campaign – which continues today – to ensure that the new benzodiazepines were brought to the attention of doctors the world over. Advertisements that appeared in medical journals on both sides of the Atlantic shamelessly demonstrated the main focus for this new generation of 'safe' medication. An article in the magazine *New Society*, entitled 'Women in a Doctored World', revealed that in advertisements for tranquillisers and antidepressants pictures of women outnumbered those of men by a ratio of fifteen to one. One such ad which was given prominence in the medical journals showed a mature woman staring into space, with tears trickling down her face. The product was Ativan – now known to many as Lorazepam. Although it is not as common now, women were generally portrayed in advertisements as emotionally weak beings in chronic need of tranquillisation; that was how Dr Douglas Porpora viewed the situation in a recent article in the *International Journal of Addiction*. Market forces, he said, lead pharmaceutical companies to promote the expanded use of tranquillisers; and particularly promoted is the prescribing of tranquillisers to women.

In her book *The Female Fix* Muriel Nellis gave some examples of the publicity hype which appeared in respected medical journals. 'MA (Fine Arts) ... PTA president elect . . . with too little time to pursue a vocation for which she has spent many years in training . . . a situation that may bespeak continuous frustration and stress'. That was a message in an advertisement for Valium. Another for Serax (Oxazepam) told doctors: 'You can't set her free. But you can help her feel less anxious. Beset by the seemingly unsurmountable problems of raising a young family and confined to the house most of the time, her symptoms reflect a sense of inadequacy and isolation.' Librium, said yet another ad, may help the older female student get back on her feet when 'afflicted by a sense of lost identity in a strange environment ... concerned over competition, apprehensive about world conditions and confronted by the possible consequences of her new freedom'.

Lyn Perry made a study of tablet use among women when she worked as information officer with the Institute for the Study of Drug Dependence in London. She too found that the medical profession's existing attitudes about women have been reinforced by the drug companies' advertising. It combined images of depressed, complaining housewives and overwrought mothers with the message that doctors can help women cope with the strains of their roles in life by relieving distress with drugs. A study was conducted among medics to determine their attitudes towards 'normal' people. They viewed 'normal healthy women' as being submissive, easily influenced, excitable – traits not in any way assigned to 'normal healthy men'. It is not surprising that twice as many women as men are prescribed benzodiazepines.

The social groups most likely to go to the doctor with anxiety or generalised discomfort are housewives, the retired and the unemployed, says Lyn Perry in her study. Further studies in Western countries had already shown that married women received twice as many prescriptions for tranquillising drugs as single women or men. But other groups in society were not immune from the clutches of the tranquilliser net. Even the young were drawn in as doctors were encouraged to prescribe to children of school age by the message that yet another brand of benzodiazepine could reduce childhood anxieties. In one ad, accompanied by the portrait of a tearful little girl, is the copyline: 'School, the Dark, Separation, Dental Visits, Monster'. The doctor is urged to help when the 'everyday anxieties of childhood sometimes get out of hand'. Some of the publicity was targeted at men, too – for instance an ad for sleeping pills bearing the comforting message: 'Normison made it with flying colours in the Falklands'.

Are doctors too easily persuaded?

In their book *Cured to Death*, Dr Arabella Melville and Colin Johnson claim that four out of every five consultations with a GP will end with the writing of a prescription for some kind of medication. Particularly where women are concerned there is a strong possibility that it will be a tranquilliser or sleeping pill. There can be no doubt that the widespread promotion of these drugs is substantially the reason for their extensive prescribing by doctors.

But Dr Heather Ashton does not believe that tranquillisers should ever be prescribed long-term for any health problem (except for people who are already dependent). Her view is that occasional short-term use for a maximum of seven to fourteen days in acute impossible anxiety situations may sometimes be necessary. The *British National Formulary* says that, although there is a tendency to prescribe benzodiazepines to almost anyone with stress-related symptoms, unhappiness or minor physical disease, their use in many situations is unjustified. The *Formulary* warns that prescribing tranquillisers to help with bereavement, for instance, may inhibit adjustment to the loss – in other words they may stop people from going through the natural and healthy process of grieving. Yet people in Liverpool were given benzodiazepines such as Lorazepam in the wake of the disaster at the Hillsborough football ground in 1989 when ninety-five football fans died.

Is it fair simply to blame the doctor? We often read about overworked GPs with long patient lists and that poses the question, is the overprescribing inevitable? My view is that doctors who issue repeat prescriptions for benzodiazepines are, in fact, mortgaging their surgery hours for years to come. In other words, an overworked GP who places patients on long-term treatment of tranquillisers or sleeping pills is likely to experience an even bigger workload later on. The most likely reason for the overprescribing of benzodiazepines is the very limited range of options available to doctors who are confronted daily with a whole range of illnesses and anxieties.

In their heyday from the swinging sixties into the seventies benzodiazepines were increasingly expected by patients, and prescribed by doctors, for almost any stress, however minor. It is hard to believe that patients would have accepted any form of medication if they had been even vaguely familiar with the potential risks. For many years these dangers were spelt out in the correspondence columns of the medical journals – to which the public did not have access, although the medical profession did. So the question who is to blame is something of a Pandora's box. Some critics say that the government regulatory bodies should have clamped down even harder when it became apparent from the numbers of prescriptions that the guidelines were largely being ignored. In the meantime, there is a lot patients can do for themselves by being firm and asking doctors and pharmacists questions about the possible side effects, addictive risks or any harmful consequences of any form of medicine offered to us.

Numerous books are now available on the subject, for example the British Medical Association has produced its own handbook for the public, the *BMA Guide to Medicines and Drugs*.

Lack of information for the public

Our organisation asked five hundred people from all over the country whether they would have ever taken a benzodiazepine if they had known what it was and 89 per cent gave a definite No. Many of these people were bitter and angry because they felt they had been lulled into the tranquilliser trap by reassuring messages from their doctor. 'They're not habit-forming', 'No, definitely not addictive', 'Take them for the rest of your life and they won't harm you', 'My wife takes them and I wouldn't give them to her if they were harmful' – these are just a few of the comforting words given out by doctors.

As Susan from Cheshire said,

I had never been a nervous type of person or depressed. I was full of beans. The doctor offered me what he described as mild muscle relaxants. They were Flurazepam (Dalmane). I felt so angry later that he made them seem so tame and harmless – how many people would associate a 'mild muscle relaxant' with what they really are: powerful brain-altering drugs?

One of the biggest-ever surveys carried out into tranquilliser use was commissioned by the popular BBC TV programme *That's Life!* After the programme's presenter, Esther Rantzen, had told viewers in graphic detail about tranquilliser withdrawal, the switchboard was jammed with other viewers wanting to tell their own stories. The survey, which was conducted in collaboration with MIND, the National Association for Mental Health, as a response to the programme, confirmed the view that very few people were ever given sufficient information about what they were being prescribed.

How ordinary people get trapped

The *That's Life! Survey On Tranquillisers*, written by Ron Lacey of *MIND* and Shaun Woodward, says that the figures pointed to the frightening statistic of 23 per cent of the British population – 10 million people – having taken tranquillisers at some time. Eighty-one per cent of the tranquilliser users who took part in the survey were women. Almost 75 per cent said they were living a contented life: most got on well with neighbours, the majority had had happy childhoods, and 60 per cent described their family homes as average. In other words, the vast majority were ordinary, normal people.

Our own mailbag over the years confirms this view; letters have poured in from professional people, teachers, nurses, managers, company directors, even doctors hooked on the tablets. The facts clearly dispute the generally accepted idea about the kind of person who takes tranquillisers. As Esther Rantzen said about her own survey: 'They are more readily identified by their normality rather than by their problems.'

In one of her projects Dr Heather Ashton listed the complaints for which patients were given their first tranquilliser or sleeping pill prescriptions; they included dizzy turns, backache, neck pain, postoperative shock, being run down, tinnitus (ringing in the ears), influenza, bereavement, anxiety and nervous problems. One woman wrote to Esther Rantzen to say that she was prescribed tranquillisers because her daughter had been made pregnant by a married man. A pensioner from Merseyside said she had first been prescribed sedatives in the early 1940s to help her cope with the German Blitz on Liverpool. She had progressed to benzodiazepines as a direct consequence of that wartime prescribing. For most people World War II is well and truly over; for this woman the battle continues – but the enemy is her tablets. What all these stories show is that ordinary people can easily receive these tablets for ordinary, everyday complaints.

The wonder drugs turn sour

Side effects

The study by the *That's Life!* team also showed that 82 per cent of the people taking part suffered side effects. The most common were panic attacks, followed by sleep problems and fear of going out of doors. Over half the people said they had first noticed the symptoms within two weeks of starting the treatment, and an incredible 90 per cent said they had not been warned to expect any reaction of this kind.

The main side effects of taking benzodiazepines are:

○ Panic attacks
○ Lack of energy and listlessness
○ Tension
○ Nervousness
○ Disturbed sleep and insomnia
○ Tiredness
○ Trembling
○ Sweating
○ Aches and pains
○ Headaches
○ Fear of going outdoors (agoraphobia)
○ Difficulty in concentrating
○ Sickness and diarrhoea.

That bald list of complaints becomes more meaningful – and more frightening – when translated into social terms. Benzodiazepines can cause oversedation which in turn can contribute to making people forgetful or careless. Their performance can suffer, which may cause problems in situations needing skill and judgement. Driving, for example, can deteriorate. Studies have shown that a large proportion of drivers involved in accidents had previously taken some form of tranquilliser. Alcohol, best avoided by drivers anyway, becomes doubly dangerous when mixed with benzodiazepines. Some tranquillisers or sleeping pills are still working the next day, so that if you are driving to work you may still be oversedated and suffering the 'hangover' effects of the tablets. Oversedation can also lead to accidents at work and in the home, and the elderly are more likely to fall and injure themselves.

Memory impairment may lead people to commit unsocial acts such as shoplifting – not because they are thieves or potential criminals, but simply because they have become forgetful. Some people can become aggressive while taking these drugs, and this can lead to domestic violence. Lost jobs, broken marriages, stained characters, children being taken into care; all these can be attributed to benzodiazepines. As one woman put it: 'I feel these tablets have robbed me of a large portion of my life.'

A *Valium* nightmare

In the mid-1970s Helen was a bright, intelligent college student studying for her degree as well as running a home. The doctor suggested that she used Valium to help her cope with her hectic life. So for two years she took the tablets without giving them a second thought. As soon as she had finished her finals Helen threw the tablets away, with her GP's full agreement.

Three days later she was plunged into an illness so severe that it shocked her family and friends: her hair was literally standing on end and she lost the use of one arm. The doctor prescribed ever more and different pills, but the woman who had been bright and breezy was turned into a human zombie. After taking an overdose she was taken to a large mental hospital. The GP turned to her husband and said, 'She'll never come out again.'

But Helen did recover, though it took time. During all the months when she was under the care of respected consultants and doctors, not once was it mentioned that her tranquillisers might have been involved in what had happened.

Over the years the memory of that dark, frightening episode continued to haunt Helen. Then, in the early 1980s, she heard me talk on a radio programme about Valium and other tranquillisers, and suddenly the pieces fell into place. She realised that the act of throwing away the tablets, with the doctor's knowledge and approval ('Yes, you won't be needing those again,' he had said), was what had plunged her into that mysterious breakdown in her mental health.

Now she is a happy, vibrant person again, highly respected in the community. Even after all these years, however, she feels angry that there is the stigma of a stay in a mental hospital in her medical records.

The warnings that went unheeded

In the same year that Helen threw away her pills, a highly respected professor joined forces with a GP to write a major warning article about benzodiazepines in the widely read *British Medical Journal*. Professor Michael Rawlins and Dr Andrew Smith, both from Newcastle, posed the question: 'Are they as safe as we think?' They observed that benzodiazepines produced psychological dependence even after short-term use, and they described how 'healthy normal' volunteers had experienced withdrawal symptoms of anxiety when they stopped taking their tablets after just two weeks. 'We know too little about the use of benzodiazepines in patients whose problems originate from intolerable social circumstances,' they wrote. They also pointed out that a survey in the 1970s had revealed that in 90 per cent of baby battering cases one parent was taking a benzodiazepine.

That was by no means the only critical article in the medical press about tranquillisers. Warnings and concerns had started to appear in the letters columns in the early 1960s, and with growing experience of the new drugs those warnings became louder and louder. Professor Malcolm Lader of the Institute of Psychiatry in London estimated that at any given moment in the late 1970s one in five women and one in ten men in the UK were taking benzodiazepines. And in the USA Barbara Gordon, an award-winning TV producer, described her battle against Valium in her bestselling autobiography *I'm Dancing as Fast as I Can*. But none of this adverse publicity made any difference to the prescribing of these wonder drugs.

What should have been the watershed for tranquillisers and sleeping pills occurred in 1980. A hard-hitting report from the British Government's Committee on the Review of Medicines (CRM) rewrote overnight the prescribing guidelines and was given extensive coverage in both the popular press and the leading medical journals: it was quite impossible for any doctor to be unaware of it.

The CRM report made it clear that the long-term

prescribing of benzodiazepines for anxiety or insomnia was inadvisable. Committee members, made up of the country's leading medical and scientific experts, had come to the conclusion that there was little evidence of the effectiveness or safety of these drugs in long-term use. They also looked at the whole question of withdrawal, and suggested that because of the problems associated with it the tablets should be withdrawn only gradually. The CRM expressed concern, too, that the similarity of withdrawal effects to the symptoms of the original illness might create a vicious circle by suggesting to doctors that the previous treatment had been inadequate, and that a further course of treatment with benzodiazepines was required. Was that the reason, the CRM wondered, why there were so many repeat prescriptions?

Until the CRM report was published there had been no specific guidelines to doctors about the duration of treatment with benzodiazepines. The CRM's conclusions were based largely on extensive research work carried out in the USA: in the late 1970s a study had been carried out by the White House Office of Drug Policy and the National Institute on Drug Abuse, culminating in a report issued by the Federal Drugs Administration in August 1979. What the committee discovered was that most of the benzodiazepine sleeping pills lost their sleep-promoting properties within three to fourteen days of continuous use. Studies had also produced little convincing evidence that tranquillisers were effective in the treatment of anxiety after four months' continuous use.

Just weeks before the CRM report sparked off new debate in British medical circles the *Observer* had run a series of articles entitled 'The Dangers of Tranquillity'. Medical correspondent Christine Doyle spoke to people who had experienced the effects of tranquillisers and who told her harrowing stories about what had happened to them when their tablets were stopped abruptly. 'How harmless is Valium?' she asked, adding: 'New facts are emerging to provide strong evidence that a substantial number of those who take it may develop physical dependence after only a few weeks on the drug.'

For some reason the message still did not seem to register, despite the avalanche of publicity. According to figures published in Hansard, the official record of proceedings in the House of Commons, prescriptions in the following year actually went up – and they increased again in 1982 and 1983! Why? One reason was that benzodiazepines were too useful for their own good: doctors had among their armoury of weapons a drug that could be given to virtually anybody for virtually everything.

During the 1980s the publicity intensified in newspapers, magazines and on television. In January 1988 a sister body to the CRM, the Committee on the Safety of Medicines (CSM), backed up the CRM's original findings and issued further prescribing guidelines to every doctor. They contained the message: '. . . withdrawal symptoms can occur with benzodiazepines following therapeutic (normal) doses given for *short* periods of time.' The Committee recommended that benzodiazepines should only be used for two to four weeks at the most, and emphasised that they were unsuitable for short-term mild anxiety.

The renewed public debate caused a number of reactions. Some doctors ignored what was said and continued to prescribe how they saw fit, others decided not to hand out any more, while yet others announced that patients taking tranquillisers were to have them withdrawn. But, as the expert committee had already pointed out, coming off these drugs posed just as many problems as staying on them.

Withdrawal symptoms – fact or fiction?

It has often been assumed that the illness caused by coming off benzodiazepines is a return to the original anxiety state. That, as pointed out in the 1980 CRM report, is not true: there is a unique and characteristic withdrawal syndrome. Sadly, a lot of people have unwittingly continued to take their tablets because of this wrong belief. 'You did need your tablets after all ... look at how anxious you are now', is the message uttered to many people by their GPs. There are three distinctive elements to the illness caused by taking, or having taken, tranquillisers and sleeping pills:

○ People may suffer from side effects from the tablets
○ They may become tolerant to the particular drug
○ They may experience withdrawal symptoms – particularly if they ignore the basic rules about taking it slowly (this is a very important point; the story of Helen – who had been wrongly advised – on p. 40 should be regarded as a cautionary tale).

Just to complicate matters, it is possible to suffer from side effects and withdrawal symptoms at the same time!
   The most commonly reported withdrawal symptoms are:

○ Anxiety
○ Insomnia
○ Nightmares
○ Panic attacks and palpitations

○ Flushing and sweating
○ Paranoid thoughts and delusions
○ Depersonalisation and feelings of unreality
○ Heightened perception of taste, smell, sound and light
○ Agoraphobia and other phobias
○ Depression
○ Poor memory and lack of concentration
○ Aggression and excitability
○ Pain, stiffness and weakness in the neck, head, jaw and limbs
○ Toothache
○ Numbness, and altered sensations in the skin (particularly in the arms, legs, mouth, jaw and tongue)
○ Muscle twitching and paraesthesia (pins and needles sensation)
○ Visual disturbance
○ Flu-type illness
○ Gastrointestinal symptoms (nausea, vomiting, abdominal pains, constipation and diarrhoea)

A lot of people undergo extensive exploratory tests and examinations in hospital because of symptoms which are not at the time associated with tablet withdrawal. Investigations for stomach problems, or neurological (e.g. brain scan) investigations, are quite common. Usually the results are negative, which means there is no physical cause for the symptoms. Some people have even been told in the past, quite wrongly, that they were suffering from multiple sclerosis. If you have experienced symptoms similar to those listed above, do remember that in all probability it was as a direct result of taking benzodiazepines. They occur in many people who have no previous history of anxiety-type symptoms.

Dr Ashton has described experiments conducted during

the 1970s on what were described as 'normal, healthy young men'. They were given benzodiazepines for just four weeks, and the tablets did indeed make them feel tranquil. But then, without them realising it, the benzodiazepines were replaced by a placebo – a dummy. For the next four weeks they experienced terrible agitation. Another group was given the sleeping pill Nitrazepam for ten days, and indeed it improved their sleep. Again, without them being aware of the fact, their pills were switched to dummy tablets, and they sufferered disturbed sleep for some time afterwards. These experiments, together with others, including one sponsored by the National Institute for Mental Health in the USA and published in *Psychopharmacology Bulletin* in 1984, show that many people, no matter how normal, experience withdrawal symptoms when their medication is stopped too quickly. These experiments were written up in medical literature in the 1970s, but nobody seems to have taken them too seriously – perhaps because the benzodiazepines were regarded as incredibly safe compared to the barbiturates which they had virtually replaced.

Some doctors still insist that patients' stated withdrawal symptoms are exaggerated, while others claim that it is really pseudo-withdrawal – patients, aware of the extensive publicity, are convinced that they will suffer and therefore imagine themselves into this situation. It seems impossible to convince some of the sceptics in the medical profession; but you should be in no doubt that these symptoms genuinely do exist.

Benzodiazepines are divided into 'long-acting' and 'short-acting' drugs – referring to the length of time that the drugs act in our bodies after we have taken them. The 1980 CRM report stated that the short-acting drugs did not tend to accumulate; this, they suggested, offered advantages in the treatment of some patients. Ironically, the majority of problems with benzodiazepines happen when these shorter-acting benzodiazepines are taken for long periods. The reason is that because of their life span in the body people who use them can experience withdrawal symptoms on a daily basis.

In a study reported in the *New England Journal of Medicine* a group of doctors closely examined what happens when benzodiazepines are withdrawn. They found that when people had taken shorter-acting benzodiazepines the symptoms started the day after the tablets had been stopped; but when people had taken long-acting tablets such as Diazepam the symptoms began to occur three to eight days after the last tablets had been taken.

Hooked before birth – tranquillisers and pregnancy

Marjorie gave birth to a healthy baby daughter. But soon after Sarah was born she started to have what appeared to be epileptic fits. The baby was taken to one of the leading children's hospitals in Britain, but the paediatricians were dumbfounded: there was no reason why Sarah should have suffered such distressing fits. Thankfully, after about nine months her attacks just stopped, and from that day until the present – she is now a teenager – she has never experienced anything remotely resembling a fit.

So what happened? It is a matter for conjecture, but there is no doubt in Marjorie's own mind (and mine) that Sarah was experiencing acute withdrawal symptoms from a benzodiazepine tranquilliser. It was only years later that Marjorie linked the fact that she had taken the drug throughout her pregnancy with the mystery fits experienced by her child.

It stands to reason when you think about it. While the baby was growing in Marjorie's womb she was getting (via her mother) a daily fix of tranquilliser. When she was born the supply was instantly stopped, so without anybody realising it Sarah went into a cold-turkey abrupt withdrawal syndrome. *The British National Formulary* states quite clearly that abrupt withdrawal may produce convulsions!

If the mother breastfeeds (Marjorie did not), abrupt withdrawal symptoms will be prevented because the child will continue to receive some of the drug through the mother's milk. But some sedative drugs can make the baby drowsy and cause feeding problems.

The sensible rule is this: if you take benzodiazepines, avoid becoming pregnant until you are off your tablets. Then make contact with a pre-conceptual care organisation (such as Foresight in England), who will give you good advice about preparing your body to ensure that the baby is healthy. After long periods on benzodiazepines this kind of advice is particularly important.

What do you do if you become pregnant while on benzodiazepines? Whatever happens, do not simply stop the medication – you must seek professional help, and insist on extra monitoring throughout your pregnancy. The Department of Psychopharmacology at Newcastle University advises the mother to get on to the lowest possible dose as soon as possible. Then, with the support of her GP, she should gradually stop taking them.

Quite apart from the withdrawal symptoms offered by the baby after birth, tranquillisers and sleeping pills can cause drowsiness in the unborn child and breathing problems at birth. In the USA, data sheets for benzodiazepines issued to doctors warn that they may damage the unborn child when taken during pregnancy. Several studies have suggested that there is an increased risk of congenital malformation if benzodiazepines are taken during the first three months: this is the most critical period when drugs may affect the developing baby.

The tranquilliser treadmill – how you get on to it, and how to keep off it

How have millions of people become trapped on tranquillisers and sleeping pills? There is a chain of events which occurs when a person embarks on a course of treatment, and you may well recognise your own situation from this.

Stage one: the first prescription. You go along to see your GP and discuss whatever problem you have. The chances are that it will be a relatively small problem or a minor physical complaint such as backache. The doctor prescribes a medicine which happens to be a benzodiazepine. Around 60 per cent of people spend less than ten minutes with their doctor during that consultation which sends them along this moving staircase of tranquilliser use. You will probably be assured that the tablets are safe and nonaddictive. At first they are effective, and do indeed instil calmness.

Stage two: the repeat prescription. Because the tablets are so effective you contact the surgery to ask for a repeat prescription. Most patients ask the receptionist to arrange this – not out of any devious motive but because they do not want to take up the doctor's valuable time. Some people can go on receiving repeat prescriptions for months or even years without ever seeing the doctor.

Stage three: the escalation of the medication. Eventually

you grow tolerant to the effects of the tablet, so the adverse side effects (which often imitate the original symptoms) start to become worse. It is also possible because of this to experience some withdrawal symptoms, even though the dosage has not been reduced. If a stressful situation occurs you need more of the drugs because by now your own control mechanism has been taken over by the benzodiazepine. So you return to the doctor, complaining that you are worse than ever and seeking help. The doctor may (a) increase the dosage, or (b) offer another benzodiazepine such as a sleeping pill. The adverse effects then start to worsen and all sorts of symptoms develop. You may, for instance, start to become agoraphobic, afraid to go out – at first you might just be reluctant to leave the house, but eventually the tablets could turn you into a virtual prisoner.

Stage four: referral to a psychiatrist. You return to the doctor, who diagnoses anxiety, phobias or whatever and refers you to a specialist – who will probably be a psychiatrist.

Stage five: the psychiatrist prescribes more drugs. You visit the specialist, and he adds antidepressants to your cocktail of drugs. Other strong tranquillising drugs may also be prescribed, and you may be sent for treatments such as behavioural therapy, cognitive therapy or hypnosis. But none of the treatments does any good because by this stage you are too heavily tranquillised. You now have an illness caused, not by anything that is wrong with you, but by the medicine. There is even a name for this condition – iatrogenic illness, which means medically induced.

So what's the next stage? Yet another nightmare trip into the downward spiral? Is this the point of no return, or can life become normal once more?

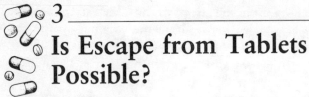

3
Is Escape from Tablets Possible?

'MY 18 YEARS OF MISERY' blared the banner headlines; 'I WAS A VALIUM PRISONER' screamed another. They tell the all too familiar story of the battle to escape from pills such as Valium and Ativan. Thousands of stories such as these appear in newspapers and magazines on both sides of the Atlantic and in every corner of the globe – the 'To Hell and Back' accounts of tranquilliser problems are legend.

But the frightening tales of people withdrawing from tablets are enough to put anybody off even considering saying goodbye to the pill that made them ill. Is it a Catch-22 situation? Or can people come off their tablets without experiencing unbearable withdrawal symptoms?

The simple answer is: yes. There *is* a safe way to escape from tranquillisers without going to Hell and back, and Part II of this book is devoted to telling you how to plan *your* safe escape from tablets, even if you have been taking them for twenty or thirty years. But first let's look at what happens to those who try to deal with the problem through what might be called normal, official channels.

When the British Government is asked to give financial support to help victims of tranquillisers, the usual answer is that the problem is well catered for by the 'drug initiative budgets'. Former MP Robert Kilroy Silk, presenter of the TV programme *Kilroy*, was among Members of Parliament who attempted to alert the Government to what he described as a drugs disaster.

While the Government is lavishing time, money and publicity on those who have made a conscious decision to use drugs like heroin, it is doing nothing or little to meet the needs and resolve the problems of those who have become dependent on a drug as a result of medical treatment and the prescribing habits of their GPs. They are addicted and in pain and distress, not because they were looking for kicks and excitement, but because they trusted their doctor.

It is questionable whether words such as 'addicted' are even accurate in relationship to benzodiazepines. These drugs are not taken for kicks; they are taken long-term because continuing them keeps away withdrawal symptoms. In the *That's Life!/MIND* survey around 95 per cent of those taking part had at some time attempted to stop taking their benzodiazepines, but well over half had resumed their tablets. As Ron Lacey, assistant director of *MIND*, commented: 'There are virtually no facilities within the health service to help people come off their tablets and deal with the horrendous withdrawal effects that occur.' The usefulness of those that do exist is debatable.

A suitable case for (hospital) treatment?

Some people feel that if they go into hospital they will be able to come off their tablets within weeks. Hospital usually means a psychiatric ward or a drug dependency unit (DDU), and such facilities would seem to be totally unsuitable for tablet withdrawal. Most users will have no previous history of mental illness – so why should they have to suffer the indignity of a psychiatric ward or, worse still, the prison-type rules applied in some drug units? Here is just a selection of the rules imposed by one such unit in Britain:

○ I will remain in night attire for seven days if staff request me to
○ I will not leave the ward without permission
○ I will provide urine or breath samples when requested
○ All activities and groups are defined as treatment and I will, therefore, attend them
○ No visitors allowed for the first week
○ No leave granted until clients have been in the unit for two weekends
○ No leave granted during the week unless for special reasons such as court attendances (presumably for drug addicts facing criminal proceedings)

Patients are warned that breaking certain rules would result in immediate discharge, uncured.

The rules of another unit demanded that drug-dependent patients had to complete 'at least three weeks in their night clothes'. They were not allowed visitors for these three weeks, and even then they could only be immediate relatives. All letters and parcels had to be opened in front of a staff member, and during the time when the patients were in their nightclothes they were not allowed to make any telephone calls. It was pointed out that the rules might vary with each individual, but many of the harsh ones were applied with vigour to some of the tranquilliser patients. Can you imagine being denied access to your family if you had a broken leg? Is there really any difference?

Ron Lacey was staggered when he read the details of these rules and regulations. 'Whilst I recognise that in the cases of opioid, barbiturate or more likely poly drug abuse, the regime described may well have relevance,' he wrote, 'from the point of view of treating benzodiazepine addicts the whole thing seems to resemble a detention centre of the "short, sharp shock" school.' The rules, he said, implied undertones of punitive authoritarianism by medical professionals who were 'resorting to the age-old defence of blaming the victim', and some of the diktats seemed almost guaranteed to humiliate the clients.

His opinion is confirmed by others in the profession. 'The regulations fill me with cold horror,' wrote a medical consultant to me, adding that DDUs are quite unsuitable for people who have 'through no fault of their own, become dependent on prescribed tranquillisers'. She made the point that tranquilliser patients form a completely different group, medically, socially and temperamentally, from alcohol and hard drug patients, and that they need gentle and sympathetic handlings, not a penal system. Referring to those rules which virtually imprison patients in DDUs, this doctor added: 'To be deprived of the support of friends and relatives just when it is needed most seems incomprehensibly cruel.'

Even if you feel that the end justifies the means, and that you can cope with these Gulag-type regimes, you may be deceiving yourself. There is no magic wand that can be waved in a hospital to enable a quick withdrawal programme to succeed. If you took note of what was written on p. 26 about the changes in the brain's 'reservoir' you will appreciate that a slow withdrawal regime is important, whether you do it at home on your own or in hospital. A slow, self-controlling programme carried out at home must surely be preferable to the potential trauma of rapid reduction in a hospital setting. A client of mine, Denise, was sent to a drug dependency unit in the north of England where she was rapidly brought off Diazepam over a couple of weeks. She still has nightmares about that experience.

Self-help groups

Many people, unable to find suitable help within the NHS (given the drawbacks, that may be a good thing), have to rely on self-help groups. In the UK there are hundreds of these groups, and many do a stirling job offering help and support to individuals. They are invariably run by former tranquilliser users, who are perhaps the best experts of all because they have 'been there'. If you find a good self-help group, count yourself fortunate, because you will be in good hands. Sadly, some groups fall by the wayside – often when the founder members become ill.

For a list of self-help groups in your area, contact your local community health council. Although many people benefit from group therapy, others prefer not to participate in this kind of approach. That wish should be respected – nobody should be forced into a group setting.

The positive alternative

If you don't like the idea of group therapy (or if your group disbands before you are completely cured), and if you don't fancy being treated like a cross between an errant schoolchild and a maximum-security prisoner, where does that leave you? Read all about my Escape Plan in Part II, and discover what thousands have found is the only safe, sensible way out of their tranquilliser predicament.

After all, going to the 'experts' won't necessarily increase your knowledge of the problem. Scientists still do not fully understand how benzodiazepines work in our bodies to achieve their main actions of controlling anxiety, relaxing muscles and helping people to sleep. In this context a wise doctor will learn from his patients, not vice versa. People who have taken benzodiazepines for years on end often know far more than the medical profession. The highest-qualified doctors in the world cannot even begin to comprehend just what it is like to take these drugs or to come off them if they have had no personal experience themselves.

The withdrawal programme has three elements:

○ *Stage one:* a healthy diet to prepare your body for the journey ahead
○ *Stage two:* a simple but effective breathing exercise that can change your whole outlook on life
○ *Stage three:* the withdrawal of tablets, showing how often and how quickly to reduce your own medication and how to work out the best and safest regime in your own individual case, using a formula

Sarah, a young woman in London who has been taking 10mg of Lorazepam (Ativan) a day, came off them with hardly any suffering. Anybody on even 3mg of Lorazepam would find that hard to believe (for reasons that we will go into later – see p. 111). But Sarah ate a lot of fresh food and salads, and also practised regular yoga during which she did a breathing control exercise. Without realising it, she had followed the advice that you are about to read in this book – and it worked perfectly.

All three stages of the plan are well recognised and respected by many leading medical authorities. Much has been written and researched about the real benefit of a correct eating pattern; the abdominal breathing was practised with incredible results at Papworth Hospital in Cambridgeshire; and the actual withdrawal regime was developed by pharmacologists at Newcastle University headed by Professor Michael Rawlins and consultant and senior lecturer Dr Heather Ashton. In this book the three stages have been merged into a single plan to give you a self-contained programme that really is the ultimate in do-it-yourself withdrawal.

First you need to take a close look at your eating habits. The chances are that if you have been on tablets for many years you will be surviving on an unhealthy diet. That is meant not as a criticism but as an acknowledgement that the tablets will probably have made you tired and lethargic, so reaching for convenience food is understandable.

Then you must learn how to breathe properly. Many users of tranquillisers and sleeping tablets hyperventilate (see p. 81), or at least breathe in the wrong way. This can easily be corrected with an effective teach-yourself programme. Of all the ways of helping yourself, this breathing method comes at the top of the list: it is the single most important step that anyone can take to help themselves achieve good health.

Incidentally, you do not even have to be a tablet user to gain a lot of benefit from the breathing exercise. It is possible that, had you been told how to perfect abdominal breathing, you would never have needed the tablets at all. It follows, therefore, that once you have completed this programme the breathing will help to make sure that you do not need tablets in the future. So stages one and two can be used as a preventative measure. They are ideal for people who have never taken tablets, and particularly for those who feel the strains and stresses of life.

The third step is the starting gate for your own withdrawal programme. It will be a long, slow process that is going to take months – nine months is the average. But don't despair at such a prospect; if you have read Chapter 2 you will appreciate the difficulties many people have found themselves in. The experience of some of those people, coupled with medical research and clinical practice, has helped in the formulation of the Escape Plan.

If you can picture a car about to enter a gruelling motor rally you will be able to appreciate the importance of all three stages. If a car is ill-prepared, the chances are it will break down or not perform well; it may even develop major faults on the journey. But by ensuring that the vehicle is in tiptop condition before the rally it is almost guaranteed an easy journey on the road ahead. Remember that you only ever want to make this journey once. You don't want to break down, and you certainly don't want to return to the starting gate. So welcome to the Escape Plan – your own chequered flag is waiting for you.

Part II
The Escape Plan

4
The Withdrawal Diet

The aim of this chapter is to convince you that a good, healthy diet is vital. Remember that your digestive system and internal organs have to process everything that is taken into your body – the food you eat, everything you drink, even the tablets you swallow. The father of medicine, Hippocrates, said over 2,500 years ago: 'Let food be your medicine'. Each one of us is born with the ability to eat, drink, breathe and rest, so looking after those four things will help us to stay well.

I do appreciate that initially it may be asking a lot for you to take on board the added burden of having to think about what you eat. Surviving from day to day may be your goal in life, and some of you will be feeling too ill to think about what you eat – indeed some of you may be hardly eating at all. Following the advice in this book unfortunately means avoiding many of the foods that people who are ill tend to rely on because of their convenience or ready availability. So please read this chapter carefully – you will quickly realise whether you are on a good diet or a bad one. The whole theme of this book is self-help, and although changing your eating patterns may at first seem an uphill struggle, I can guarantee that you will be well rewarded for your efforts.

Doctors are not nutritionists

Dr Peter Mansfield is a GP working in Lincolnshire. But unlike many members of his profession Dr Mansfield carefully assesses the diet and eating patterns of his patients when they seek his help. In *The Good Health Handbook* he says people should realise that doctors do not in general understand nutrition, having been taught very little about it during their days at medical school.

Ideas about nutritional therapy, he says, have been opposed with irrational hostility by the medical profession. Many doctors have even had the opportunity of trying nutritional medicine themselves and seeing the results, but still the message is largely ignored. The reason, Dr Mansfield suggests, is this: 'In the absence of any other explanation for this from doctors themselves we may suppose that ideas like these [nutritional medicine] are too cheap, too successful and too little dependent on professional help to win medical approval.' Diet as a method of treatment completely undermines the doctors' own time-honoured basis of medicine. But their method, he adds, diminishes in significance like a punctured balloon when diet is seen to prevent and even cure most, if not all, disease.

Try to think of it in this way. For years many of you will have had your lives controlled by tranquillisers or sleeping pills, probably on a daily basis. For supplies of those tablets you have had to rely on the doctor – there is little you can do about that. Medicines offered by the doctor, be they liquid, tablets or capsules, are designed to offer relief from symptoms – they do not provide a cure. The curing is left to you and your body, so why not follow the immortal words of Hippocrates and let food be *your* medicine?

In a recent book on the subject of Oriental medicine, Daniel Reid discussed the question of mental health and diet. 'Psychoanalysis as practised in Western medical circles does not exist in the traditional Chinese medical system. When a patient in the Orient displays symptoms of emotional stress, mental confusion, panic attacks, paranoia, the truly good physician first tries to cure it by food.' And in *Nutrition and Your Mind*, Dr George Watson of the University of California says that psychiatrists attach great importance to a whole range of mental symptoms such as depression, mania and neurosis when in fact the symptoms were usually caused by severe nutritional imbalance and behaviour. He sums up the whole message by saying: 'What you eat determines your state of mind and who you are.'

Natural food is better, raw food is best

Healthy eating, said Dr Malcolm Carruthers, is a timeless science, researched for thousands of years in different civilisations but surprisingly neglected in the twentieth century. He expressed that sentiment in a foreword to one of my favourite books, *Raw Energy*, by Leslie and Susannah Kenton. Leslie and her daughter are known throughout the world for their advice about healthy eating, and they recommend plenty of raw food – 75 per cent of what we eat should consist of raw food, which they describe as the Mind Lift.

Susannah used to suffer from bouts of depression for no obvious reason. After several weeks on a high raw food diet they stopped; however, it only took a weekend of old-style eating to bring back one of her familiar lows. With a diet high in raw food they both found they were much more even tempered and clear-thinking. 'That makes us wonder if many of the negative feelings we all get from time to time are not so much psychological in origin as physiological, a sign that body chemistry is out of balance and toxins are building up,' they say. That is precisely the message I have been hammering home for years – that there are physical reasons for psychological symptoms. It follows that the solution is to adjust your own body chemistry to get rid of the symptoms.

But the question they pose is: why should a regime of raw food make us feel so different? Why should people eating lots of raw food find themselves better able to cope with chronic fatigue, irritability and lethargy, which they describe as the plague of modern civilisation?

The answer, in general terms, is that many of the nutrients crammed into vegetables, fruit and other fresh food are essential for a healthy nervous system. To put it another way, cooking and refining destroy much of the nutritional value in our food. Stephen Davies and Dr Alan Stewart have shown that a diet consisting mainly of processed or refined foods is often deficient in magnesium, one of the body's most important minerals. Interestingly, they say in their book *Nutritional Medicine*, the same symptoms as those of magnesium deficiency can be observed in neuropsychiatric disorders. Just look at some of the symptoms they list as resulting from magnesium deficiency:

○ Apathy
○ Depression
○ Nervousness
○ Anxiety
○ Weakness and tiredness
○ Numbness and tingling

○ Confusion and disorientation
○ Memory impairment
○ Vertigo
○ Muscle cramps
○ Tremors
○ Insomnia
○ Hyperactivity
○ Constipation
○ Heart rhythm problems
○ Premenstrual tension.

In fact the two doctors say that people displaying any of these symptoms should be checked for magnesium deficiency. Has your doctor ever suggested to you an assessment of your magnesium level?

So where can you find magnesium, apart from supplements bought over the counter in a health shop or pharmacy? Green leafy vegetables are one of the best-known sources – the greener the vegetable, the more magnesium. Other rich sources are nuts, whole grains, shrimps and soya beans. No wonder the Kentons' high raw food diet made them much more resistant to stress!

When they questioned experts about the reasons for this, they learned that it was probably due to the way in which raw foods affect the body's alkaline balance. 'Balanced body chemistry is not merely a recipe for keeping calm and collected, but a fundamental necessity for health,' they say, adding that overaccidity in the body lies at the root of many illnesses.

What does this alkalinity/acidity mean? Virtually all the food we eat has an acid-forming or alkaline-forming effect. If your diet contains a lot of sugar, coffee, meat and other concentrated proteins, and processed foods made from white flour (but only small quantities of fresh vegetables and fruit), you are consuming mainly acid foods and you will tend to feel stressed very easily. A combination of acid-forming foods and periods of stress sends the body's acid levels up and up, so the antidote to stress is to eat plenty of alkaline-forming foods. The suggested ratio is four to one, which means that ideally 80 per cent of the food you eat needs to be alkaline-forming, and when you are exposed to stressful situations the level needs to be even higher. Good alkaline foods are:

○ Dried fruit (apricots, figs, prunes, raisins, currents, sultanas and peaches)
○ Dates
○ Almonds and brazil nuts
○ Chestnuts
○ All vegetables (but especially avocados, beetroot and spinach)
○ Fruit and berries
○ Milk.

All meat, fish and shellfish, cheese and eggs are high acid-formers. So when you eat these foods it is a good idea to ensure a good balance by also eating plenty of alkaline-forming foods.

Another advocate of a high alkaline diet is Celia Wright, author of the highly popular *Wright Diet*. 'You can spend a lifetime trying to get to the bottom of your problems,' she says, 'psychotherapy, astrology, Harley Street doctors – the list is endless. Yet I sometimes wonder if this simple principle of diet hasn't got as much to offer as the best of them.' Eating the correct food is the surest way of controlling the alkaline level of our blood – we have the choice of being relaxed or irritable, says Celia. The most immediate experience of eating a diet containing 80 per cent alkaline-forming foods is one of overwhelming well-being, calmness, emotional stability, strength without aggression and a constant feeling of optimism, she adds. She suggests that psychiatrists and sociologists are going to have to take notice of this vital dietary factor.

Clearly this kind of diet is food for us all, but during tablet withdrawal it is vital. Susan was finding it so hard to come down off her tablets. She was getting little or no support from her family doctor, her husband did not understand her problems, and she felt tired and edgy most of the time: the least thing would upset her, so she was constantly in tears. Her lack of energy meant that she was living on a really bad diet: toast, biscuits, cakes, tea and coffee. She did not have the energy to prepare, let alone cook, decent food.

But eventually the message got home and slowly she started to make herself eat more salads and then more vegetables, both cooked and raw. It did not take long for her quality of life to take a quantum leap forward. She is now off her tablets, living a normal, happy life, and even slowly converting the rest of the family to her way of eating. It was an amazing transformation – just a few months before she had been a physical and nervous wreck. The important thing was that Susan continued to eat healthily even after stopping her tablets.

What is a healthy diet?

Although some kinds of food have been pinpointed as causing problems, that does not mean you should stop eating them altogether. A healthy diet is always a balanced diet. Follow these general rules:

○ Eat as little processed or refined food as you can
○ Remember to keep up the level of alkaline-forming food
○ Go for raw food whenever possible.

A bonus of eating a diet based on natural foods is that you will shed unwanted pounds effortlessly.

Foods and drinks to avoid

I am afraid, however, that eating healthily means a fond farewell to what may be some of your favourites:

○ White bread
○ Cakes
○ Biscuits
○ Any other food made with white flour
○ Refined or polished (white) rice
○ Chocolate, sweets and sugary foods
○ Sugary drinks
○ Caffeine-containing drinks (tea, coffee and cola).

Unless you can be absolutely sure of the ingredients, tinned or packeted foods are best avoided. The trouble with tea and coffee is that their caffeine content can keep you awake, particularly at bedtime. It can continue working in your body for something like six hours, so if you have tea or coffee at 6 p.m. it is still working around midnight.

It may surprise many people, but giving up tea or coffee is easier said than done: there is a possibility of withdrawal symptoms if caffeine intake is stopped suddenly. It is much better to cut down to between two and four cups of weak tea a day and gradually phase it out altogether; in any case avoid tea or coffee after about 6 p.m.

Alcohol should be avoided totally if you are using tranquillisers or sleeping pills. Benzodiazepines are more harmful when mixed with alcohol.

Aim to eat fresh (not canned or processed) meat, fish, vegetables and fruit. Wholegrains only should be used – particularly wholemeal bread, wholegrain brown rice and wholewheat pasta. Many people like the comforting texture of hot cooked vegetables, but we should also aim to eat at least one bowlful of mixed raw vegetables each day. Green leafy vegetables such as spinach, lettuce and cabbage are particularly good. The healthy nutrients will act as a real tonic for your body as you prepare for that all-important journey ahead.

What about drinking? Fresh fruit juices are fine, along with good-quality bottled or filtered tap water. For a healthy hot drink try herbal teas. Limeflower and camomile are useful natural relaxants, so can be drunk at bedtime.

Tips on healthy foods

○ Did you know that lettuce is regarded as a natural tranquilliser? It contains a chemical called lactucin which helps to induce a state of relaxation

○ Raw cabbage is packed with vitamin C, one of the most important vitamins

○ Cucumbers and string beans are rich in potassium, one of the most important minerals

○ Grapes help to detoxify the body and are good for instant energy. Black grapes are best

○ Sunflower seeds are a good source of nutrients such as iron, vitamin E and the nervous system's favourite combination, the B vitamins. These seeds have a sedating effect. It is a good idea to keep a supply in your handbag or pocket as an emergency snack. Add a few pumpkin seeds for variety

○ Beetroot helps menstrual problems. Grated or chopped, it adds taste and colour to a mixed salad

○ The carrot has been called the best therapeutic food in the world: this vegetable really is an antidote for stress. Eat it raw or drink carrot juice (make your own or buy it from health-food shops). Nibble on carrot sticks as a snack

○ Celery contains a good helping of minerals

○ Pecan nuts are one of the best-known sources of natural pyridoxine (vitamin B6)

○ Bananas are packed with healthy minerals such as potassium and magnesium. They are also rich in tryptophan, one of the amino acids, which helps promote restful sleep

○ Turkey is also packed with tryptophan. A turkey sandwich (or a banana sandwich) is a great late-night snack

○ Porridge oats, popular in Scotland, are an underrated health food. They are in fact one of the best tonics for the body's nervous system. They help build stamina and energy and have also been credited with helping depression. They can be eaten as a breakfast cereal or used to make biscuits

○ Wheatgerm oil is a good source of vitamin E

○ Mangoes have qualities which help deal with depression.

How to survive on a healthy diet!

Start each day with a glass of room-temperature clean water half an hour an hour before breakfast. Then make sure you eat a healthy breakfast, such as porridge oats or some other cereal with fruit. Look at the ingredients on labels and avoid those with added sugar or other additives. Wash your fruit well, especially if it isn't organically grown.

For the rest of the day you may find it easier to eat little and often – say every three hours. This will balance your blood sugar level, which is important when you are withdrawing from tablets. You won't be eating more – just spreading your daily quota of food over five or six snack meals. It is usually a good idea to have one of these snack meals at bedtime to keep your blood sugar level even while you are asleep. Remember that a turkey or banana wholemeal sandwich is ideal at bedtime, perhaps with a glass of warm milk.

Other simple but healthy snacks include sliced banana on rye crispbread, or sugar-free jam on wholemeal bread. Don't forget pulses such as lentils, and sprouted seeds and beans such as alfalfa, mung, aduki and chick peas. Sprouted food contains large amounts of nutrients and it is very simple to grow at home.

If you cannot face the thought of raw veg, try eating just a little alongside your favourite cooked vegetable and gradually increase the amount. Another idea is to cook a casserole containing meat and vegetables and to pour the hot cooked food over a portion of raw vegetables. If you say you are too ill to eat this kind of food it probably means you need to eat it more than anybody.

Try to eat plenty of fish, particularly deep-sea fish such as cod and haddock. If you do eat beef, pork or lamb try not to have large portions. Gradually you will work out your own ideas, and I hope that this chapter will act as a springboard to help you control your health in the future. A few simple recipes are given on p. 74 just to show how easy it can be to start on a healthier way of eating. I see food as the great liberator of us ordinary people who in the past have had to rely on doctors to supply cures (!) for our ailments. With food we can control what we take into our mouths and become responsible for ourselves.

Vitamin and mineral supplements

One of the main reasons why a healthy natural diet is advocated during tablet withdrawal is because it is packed with nutrients. During a five-month campaign on BBC television a doctor advocated the use of good vitamin and mineral supplements at this time, and in *The Wright Diet* respected nutritionist Celia Wright suggests that people coming off tranquillisers should take daily multi-vitamin and multi-mineral tablets as well as vitamin C. Whether or not you take supplements is something you should discuss with your own medical adviser. It is far better to get professional guidance than just to take all kinds of vitamins and supplements.

Simple recipes

These are a few of my own favourites which are quick and easy to prepare.

Raw vegetable salad (Serves 1–2)

1–2 tomatoes
1 medium carrot
¼ cabbage
1 medium onion

1–2 spring onions
1–2 spinach leaves
2–3 lettuce leaves
2 cauliflower florets
¼ cucumber
1 stick of celery
4oz/125g sprouted seeds and beans such as mung or
  alfalfa (available ready-grown in health stores and
  some supermarkets)
1 dessertspoon sunflower seeds (optional)
1 dessertspoon pumpkin seeds

Thoroughly wash the vegetables under running water.
Cut them into small pieces or shred them in a food
processor. Place the vegetables in a glass bowl and cover
with clingfilm. Place in the refrigerator, and whenever
you eat a meal or snack have a few spoonfuls of this
raw vegetable salad which is crammed with healthy
nutrients.

Green vegetable salad (Serves 1–2)

2–4 lettuce leaves
¼ cabbage
1–2 spinach leaves
1–2 Chinese cabbage leaves
1 medium onion *or* 1 bunch spring onions

Slice or shred the green vegetables, then chop the onion
and add it. Ideal as a side salad when eating hot meals.

Hot and cold casserole (Serves 2)

8–12oz/250–350g beef *or* lamb (use ready-minced if
 you like)
1 medium onion
2 tablespoons cooking oil (cold-pressed is best)
6oz/175g marrowfat peas (soaked overnight)
6oz/175g red *or* green *or* brown lentils (or a mixture)
2–3 carrots
1 small to medium turnip
2 leeks
Black pepper to taste
Pinch of salt

Trim any fat from the meat and if necessary cut it into
small cubes (a good butcher will gladly do this for you if
requested). Chop the onion, and gently fry the meat and
onion in the oil. Place the lentils and marrowfat peas in
a large pan of water and bring to the boil. Leave on a
high temperature for 10 minutes, then reduce the heat
and simmer them. Dice the carrots, turnips and leeks,
and add them to this pan along with the meat and
onions. Continue to cook on a low heat for at least an
hour, stirring occasionally. Add pepper and salt. The
peas or lentils will act as a thickener to make a really
wholesome, simple casserole.

To serve, place a quantity of mixed raw vegetables or
green raw vegetables (see the previous two recipes) on a
plate and top with a portion of hot casserole.

Onion soup (Serves 2)

1lb/500g onions
1lb/500g potatoes
1½ pints/900ml water
1 stock cube
1 bouquet garni
1 tablespoon wholewheat flour *or* cornflour
Salt
Black pepper

Chop the onions and potatoes, then simmer for about 30 minutes in the water to which the stock cube and bouquet garni have been added. Place the flour in a bowl and stir in a small quantity of cold water to slake it. To this mix add about half the partly cooked soup, stirring well to avoid lumps forming. Pour this mixture into the pan containing the rest of the soup. Stir occasionally. Continue to heat for about 10–15 minutes, but do not let the soup boil. Remove the bouquet garni before serving.

Simple pea and ham soup (Serves 2)

1lb/500g marrowfat peas (soaked overnight)
6oz/175g ham *or* gammon
1 medium to large onion
1 leek
1 carrot
Salt
Black pepper
¼ teaspoon tumeric
1 beetroot (raw)

Drain the liquid off the peas, put them in a large pan and cover with water. Dice the ham, onion, leek and carrot, add them to the pan and leave on medium heat for 20 minutes. Reduce the heat to a simmer, stirring occasionally. Add the salt, pepper and tumeric. Grate the beetroot and garnish the soup with it.

Beans with cauliflower (Serves 2)

1 cauliflower
1 tablespoon cold-pressed oil *or* ½oz/15g margarine
1 medium onion
12oz/350g haricot beans, dried *or* tinned (soaked overnight if dried)

Cut the cauliflower into large florets and place them in a pan of water. Cook for about 10 minutes until tender but not soft. In a frying pan gently melt the margarine or oil. Chop the onion and add it to the pan along with the haricot beans. Gently fry until the beans are heated through. Place the cauliflower in a serving dish and top with the fried haricot beans. Serve with a green salad.

Simple oatcakes (Serves 2)

8oz/250g porridge oats
2oz/60g fine oatmeal
1 cup filtered water
Banana *or* apple *or* pineapple *or* sultanas *or* fresh or dried apricots (optional)

Preheat the oven to 180°C (350°F/gas mark 4). Mix the oats, oatmeal and water to a firm consistency in a bowl. Add fresh or dried fruit as desired, chopped if necessary. Take small amounts of the mixture and place on a greased baking tray to make biscuit-sized oatcakes. Alternatively use a round pastry cutter. Bake for 15–20 minutes.

Eat hot or cold, topped with natural yoghurt, as a healthy snack. Carry a few with you when you are out as a good emergency snack.

Variations: Use a mixture of grains to add variety, and cook in the same way.

Fruit salad (Serves 2)

1 apple
1 pear
1 banana
4–6oz/125–175g grapes
½ orange
1 slice pineapple
1 kiwi fruit
1 peach
2 apricots
Selection of dried fruit
1 teaspoon lemon juice *or* freshly squeezed orange
   juice

Thoroughly wash all the fruit. Peel, slice and cut into chunks as appropriate, mix together and add the juice. Serve topped with a small carton of natural yoghurt.

Yoghurt with nuts (Serves 1)

1 tablespoon mixed seeds and nuts (e.g. sunflower
  seeds, pumpkin seeds, hazelnuts, brazil nuts,
  pecans)
6–8 sultanas
1 carton natural yoghurt
1 small banana, sliced (optional)

Mix the seeds, nuts and sultanas into the yoghurt for a
healthy instant snack or pudding. If desired, top with
sliced banana.

Emergency snack

An even blood sugar level is crucial during withdrawal.
When you go out shopping or for an evening carry a
bag of mixed nuts, sunflower seeds and dried apricots
and dip into it as and when required – far better than
rushing into the nearest shop for a bar of chocolate!

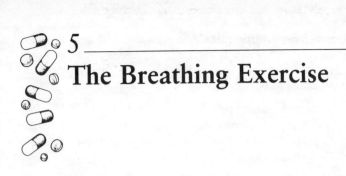

5
The Breathing Exercise

This chapter describes what is the single most important aid to withdrawing from tablets. The breathing exercise is simple, effective and will help to control or even eliminate many of the more common withdrawal symptoms such as panic attacks, palpitations and rapid heartbeat. We all breathe – it is a necessary function of the body, and when we stop breathing permanently we die. Because it is a vital function of the body it is controlled automatically – without us having to think or worry about it. We breathe while we work, eat, sleep, pursue leisure activities. But what we can control is the *way* we breathe.

Hyperventilation and tranquillisers

Over the years it has been my experience and that of others working in this area of health that many users of tranquillisers and sleeping pills breathe in the wrong way – they hyperventilate. While it is not dangerous or life-threatening, it can cause a whole range of physical and psychological symptoms that make life at best uncomfortable and at worst intolerable.

Hyperventilation means that you are breathing in the wrong way, usually taking breaths into your upper chest. You can clearly see many people hyperventilating because their chests move quite quickly as they breathe in and out. In others, though, it is not so obvious, and a lot of people are themselves unaware that they are breathing incorrectly.

This problem has a special relevance for people taking benzodiazepines, since one of the functions of these drugs is that of a muscle relaxant. But included in the muscular system, and therefore susceptible to the effects of the drug, are the muscles that control our breathing. So it is not at all surprising that breathing patterns go haywire after long-term use of benzodiazepines and particularly when people come off them too quickly. The process of coming off tablets can temporarily heighten this muscular effect, causing some people to become even more panicky or to experience palpitations. Learning how not to hyperventilate is therefore crucial to your eventual full recovery.

Why do people hyperventilate?

Hyperventilation, wrote physiotherapist Rosemary Cluff in the *Journal of the Royal Society of Medicine*, is a perfectly normal reaction to stress. Most of us at some time during our lives will have experienced the classic signs of hyperventilation during stressful situations or in a crisis – the racing heart or the butterflies in the stomach. But in normal circumstances, once the situation is over the symptoms will lift.

However, many people hyperventilate not only during periods of stress but all the time. There is no particular reason why people breathe incorrectly on a permanent basis. It would seem to be simply a habit built up over many years, possibly a lifetime. I strongly suspect that a great number of people were hyperventilating long before they were ever prescribed tablets, and that the incorrect breathing pattern was the reason for their journey into the world of tranquillisers. So if an individual had been 'prescribed' breathing lessons instead of a brain-altering medicine would it have been better? Without hesitation I would reply: yes! Miss Cluff worked with chest consultant Dr Claud Lum at Papworth Hospital in Cambridgeshire, where they achieved remarkable results among ill people by teaching them how to stop hyperventilating.

Symptoms caused by hyperventilation

There are a great many symptoms caused by hyperventilation and they can affect any part of the body, though there are some almost universal symptoms suffered by hyperventilators:

- General exhaustion
- Lack of concentration
- Diminished performance
- Sleep disturbance
- Nightmares
- Emotional sweating.

Here are just some of the other symptoms that can be caused by breathing in the wrong way:

- Blackouts
- Palpitations
- Heart pains
- Missed heartbeats
- Dizziness
- Faintness
- Visual disturbances

○ Pins and needles, particularly of the hands, feet and face
○ Irritable cough
○ Heartburn
○ Gastrointestinal problems
○ Muscular cramps
○ 'Fibrositis' of the neck, back or shoulders
○ Tension and anxiety
○ Unreal feelings
○ Fear of insanity
○ General fatigue
○ Physical weakness
○ Exhaustion
○ Lack of concentration and memory
○ Depersonalisation
○ Hallucinations
○ Migrainous headache
○ Numbness.

If you suffer a number of these symptoms, there is a very strong possibility that you are hyperventilating.

Interestingly, one perception which is not heightened by hyperventilation is pain. The complex sensation recognised as pain is dulled or abolished, and sometimes it is just as well! During ritual mutilation ceremonies in tribal initiation or voodoo rites the excitement, singing, dancing and beating of drums induce a crescendo of hyperventilation during which initiates are able to endure what would otherwise be extremely painful procedures.

It is little wonder, says Dr Lum, that patients with the symptoms listed above are usually regarded as neurotic. Some people even keep the symptoms to themselves, thinking that they will be regarded as 'going mad'. Because the symptoms of hyperventilation can so easily be misunderstood by doctors, a lot of patients are sent to clinics and hospitals to undergo a whole range of expensive tests. It is not uncommon for a person to have heart investigations or gastrointestinal checks which will invariably be fruitless. Instead of getting help the patient acquires a thick medical file, which tends to add even more to those unfair labels of 'neurotic' or 'nuisance'. Many of you reading this will recognise the chain of events only too well.

It is a great pity that doctors do not consider the possibility of hyperventilation more carefully, given that they are unable to explain the cause for symptoms in at least one-third of patients seeking their help. Sadly, there is a tendency to apply the blanket diagnosis 'neurosis' or 'anxiety state' to cover the inability of some doctors to explain why patients suffer from multiple symptoms for which no obvious cause can be found. So there is a strong temptation to write out a prescription for benzodiazepine tranquillisers, sleeping pills or some other pharmaceutical from the family of anxiety-cum-sedative drugs.

Some members of the profession have, however, seen the light. Recently, respected professor of psychiatry Sydney Brandon wrote an article telling family doctors how to handle depression among their patients. Before giving out antidepressants, he advised, the GP should check the breathing to discover whether the patient is hyperventilating. This was one of those rare occasions on which a doctor recognised the possibility of physical causes for depression.

Does anxiety cause the symptoms, or is it the other way around? Opinions vary, but many doctors, including Dr Lum, insist that it is hyperventilation that causes anxiety. To demonstrate the point he cites a number of interesting examples. Hyperventilation can be triggered off by a purely physical illness, or by a general anaesthetic before an operation. Somebody who exhibits a driving personality at work will often suffer the first attack of hyperventilation at the weekend or on holiday. It can even be sparked off by something as simple as a change of mood, happiness, laughter, relief or watching television. The point he makes is that anxiety then develops out of the symptoms brought on by hyperventilating.

In 1950 an American doctor studied incorrect breathing and came to the same conclusion. He also found that the anxiety could be cured by eliminating faulty breathing habits. That experience was confirmed by Dr Lum and Miss Cluff among their patients at Papworth Hospital, most of whom were generally classified on arrival as neurotic or suffering from anxiety states, anxiety-depression, panic disorders or similar problems.

Over 1,500 patients received a course in breathing retraining and relaxation in the physiotherapy department, and their symptoms usually went in a matter of months. Some of the younger patients were cured within weeks, while some of the older or more severe cases took some months. Twelve months after the treatment started, 75 per cent were completely free of all symptoms and 20 per cent were left with occasional or mild symptoms which did not trouble them.

How to do the crucial breathing exercise

Known as the Papworth Breathing Exercise, this is the same one taught for a number of years by Dr Lum, Miss Cluff and their staff.

1. Lie down on the floor, or on a bed, with your head on a cushion or book. Try generally to relax your body if

you can. Your legs can be either straight or bent at the knees, but do not cross your legs or ankles.

2. Place one hand on your chest and the other hand on your stomach.
3. Take a nice, long, slow breath inwards and watch your hands. The hand placed on your chest should not move at all, but the one placed on your stomach should rise as though you are inflating a balloon.
4. Hold your breath for a second or so, and then breathe out just as slowly as you breathed inwards.
5. Continue with this exercise for fifteen to thirty minutes and do it at least twice a day, for example mid-morning and early evening. A few minutes' abdominal breathing in bed at night will also be a big help.
6. During the day be aware of your breathing without becoming obsessive about it. Think about the way you breathe for just a minute every hour.
7. If you wish, play some music to help you relax while doing the breathing exercise.
8. The aim is for your breathing (from the abdomen) to become silent and effortless.
9. Once you have perfected abdominal breathing in the lying position, progress to practising the exercise sitting, standing and even walking – aiming always to keep a slow, steady breathing rhythm.

It is a very simple and straightforward exercise, but even so the chances are that many people will not be able to breathe like that immediately. Many of you will notice that, when you place your hands on your stomach and chest, the wrong one, or both, moves up and down. Please be patient and continue to practise – the rewards are far too great to ignore!

When I first devised my Escape Plan the doctor who

vetted it for me suggested that the breathing exercise should also be done by people who have never used tranquillisers, as a means of looking after their health. So it is good idea for couples – say, for instance, a wife who uses tablets and her husband (or vice versa) to practise this exercise together.

How long should the breathing exercises be practised before embarking on a tablet withdrawal regime?

This will vary with each individual, but as a rule of thumb it is much better to ensure that you are perfectly happy with your breathing pattern before starting a reduction programme. On average it is going to take about six weeks of twice daily practice. Some people will need to take longer, but it is well worth the time and trouble taken to perfect this exercise. Some people, eager to withdraw from their tablets, decide to change their diet, learn the breathing and start the withdrawal programme all at once. For most people that is far too much to handle. Patience will be well rewarded if the breathing and diet are attended to well in advance of any withdrawal regime. If after six weeks of regular practice your breathing is still not correct you will need to continue with the exercises and perhaps consider seeking the professional help of a physiotherapist.

Help from a physiotherapist

You could ask your own doctor to arrange a hospital referral to a physiotherapist, but you are unlikely to be successful, since there is a chronic shortage of these people and their time is valuable. Many, however, are in private practice (look in Yellow Pages or the Business Section of your telephone directory) and will give lessons in abdominal breathing – though you will, of course, have to pay. It is well worth it – you may only need a handful of sessions to get you into the swing of things, and lasting good health is priceless.

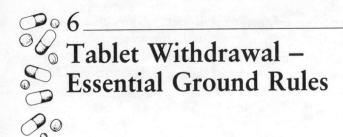

6

Tablet Withdrawal – Essential Ground Rules

Finally, after learning how to breathe properly and having cleansed your system through following a sensible, healthy diet, you can start planning your withdrawal from tranquillisers. This chapter explains the general rules that apply to all the medications covered in Chapters 7–10 – don't skip it in your haste to get on to the chapter dealing with your own particular tablet.

Make your own decisions

The first thing to get clear in your mind is that you, the patient, are in the best position to make three major decisions:

1. Whether you want to come off tablets after long-term use
2. How quickly you should withdraw
3. By what amounts you should withdraw.

Only you know exactly how much stress and strain there is in your life at any given moment. For many people there will never be an ideal time to start a withdrawal programme. But the knowledge that you will be able to cut down at a rate *you* feel happy with is a great help. Knowing that a doctor will not hurry you along is more likely to ensure that you embark on and stick to a withdrawal regime. It is so important for reduction plans to be a two-way thing between the patient and doctor. Self-motivation is vital, and experience shows that many people are genuinely motivated to escape from their tablets, if only they knew how to do it. However, there seems little or no point in dragging somebody off tablets if they do not want to come off them. Any doctor who does so is guaranteed to be bombarded with visits and requests for home calls from potentially ill sufferers.

Unfortunately, there are still some doctors around today who tell people to stop instantly, despite the dangers, and who impose a withdrawal regime unilaterally and instruct the patient to get on with it. 'If you are going to come off them, let's get it over and done with', is a phrase uttered all too often. Doctors, it would appear, do this for no other reason than that they believe they are doing the right thing. Most will assume they are acting in the best interests of the patient: some no doubt honestly believe that by giving a laid-down, rigid programme they are actually doing the patient a big favour. But thousands of people have written to me to say that they have been terrified when deadlines or target dates have been stipulated.

Not so long ago there was an avalanche of panic calls to our office from people in one particular town in Cheshire. Their GP had made it known that his New Year's resolution was not to prescribe any more tranquillisers. His message to patients was: enjoy your Valium, Ativan, Mogadon or whatever at Christmas, because by the New Year there will be no more. After some diplomatic prodding he broke his resolution even before the old year was out. But it did cause unnecessary heartache and avoidable misery at what should have been a joyous time.

Simon, in his mid-twenties, telephoned from London – in tears. His mother had been taking a tranquilliser for years, but without notice or warning the GP had suddenly decided there would be no more tablets. He would not listen to any pleas or requests from Simon or his sisters, who watched their mother growing daily more ill. A courteous and diplomatic telephone call to the surgery was made to point out the problem, reinforcing the view that gradual withdrawal was essential. The doctor listened, though he was somewhat resentful about interference from an outside lay organisation. Within a few hours Simon's mother had her medication restored and the family set about helping her off her tablets in the way outlined in this book.

Contrast those stories with a letter received as this chapter was being written early in 1990. It was from a lady in Northamptonshire, who a year ago embarked on my Escape Plan to come off Lorazepam.

I have been meaning to write ever since to say just how marvellous I found the advice in your plan. It was invaluable in helping me to understand just what was going on, and probably more than anything was very reassuring that if one did cut down slowly enough one wouldn't experience the terrifying withdrawal symptoms that I had experienced. It really is possible to escape from Lorazepam, even if you don't feel you have the support of your GP or family.

Thankfully, a growing number of doctors are now recognising what workers in this area of health have been saying for years – that it is the patient who should decide if, when and how. Do discuss things calmly with the doctor. If you decide that you want to have a go at coming off the tablets, tell your GP, ask for support and encouragement, and stress that you need to do it at a rate you feel comfortable with. If you have been getting limitless repeat prescriptions for years on end, ask for a reasonable supply; you do not, for instance, want the tablets to be suddenly rationed. Knowing that you have enough for any emergency is comforting during a withdrawal programme. Tell the doctor that if he or she agrees with your plan and accepts what you say about cutting down slowly, you are far more unlikely to be a burden on the surgery. That, of course, is a massive plus for the GP!

Meanwhile, here are answers to some of the questions we are most frequently asked by people considering the possibility of coming off tranquillisers.

I like the idea of a slow withdrawal regime similar to the one you have outlined. But my doctor says that withdrawal symptoms are all in the mind and caused by all the publicity. He says if I stop reading about the problem I won't suffer.

If that was true, many people would gladly call for a total ban on publicity about tranquilliser withdrawal. But you would be amazed at the number of people who have never realised that they were taking a tranquilliser or sleeping pill. Glance through some of the brand names in this book – unless you are an expert in pharmaceuticals how could you ever have been expected to realise that they were benzodiazepines and related to perhaps the best-known one, Valium. The interesting thing is that when people unaware that their medication was from this family dumped their tablets, they became ill. Clearly that could not be attributed to the psychological effects of heavy publicity.

I am a sensible man with a high-powered job and feel I have not got the time to follow a slow programme such as the one you advocate. I do not feel that I am the type to suffer from withdrawal symptoms.

It would be nice if we could determine in advance those at risk of symptoms and those who will sail through the whole thing and wonder what all the fuss is about. But unfortunately nobody really knows what type of person will suffer from symptoms. It is much better to be patient, take your time and avoid any possible suffering. Professor Malcolm Lader has warned that the withdrawal symptoms are not always helped by resuming benzodiazepine treatment – yet another good reason for slow withdrawal.

If I do suffer from any withdrawal symptoms, how long will they last?

If there was a league table of questions most often asked, this would be at the top of the list. Some books and some counsellors have stated that symptoms last for a given number of weeks or months, depending on the length of time the tablets were taken. There is no justification for such equations at all. One distressed woman had worked out that her own symptoms were due to last seven months, three weeks and two days; then she wondered why she did not wake up after seven months, three weeks and three days feeling 100 per cent well.

The simple answer is that nobody knows, and there is no scientific or mathematical basis for working out accurately the duration of withdrawal. Some people can come off tablets after twenty years' or more use with relative ease; others suffer symptoms after just a few weeks on the tablets. At the end of the day it all must depend on the state of your general health, as well as ensuring that you follow an extremely slow withdrawal regime. The breathing plan and diet outlined in Chapters 4 and 5 are designed to place you in the best possible position for a trouble-free withdrawal.

Are there any tablets I can take to ease withdrawal symptoms?

The simple answer is no, except perhaps for something more powerful and potent than the tranquilliser currently being used. But that would be self-defeating, for it would be likely to create even bigger problems in the future. For specific symptoms some doctors will prescribe occasional painkillers, or will give beta-blockers or antidepressants to help with tremors, palpitations or depression. But the majority of people prefer to plan their withdrawal programme without other medication.

One safe form of help is the Bach Flower Remedies, devised in the 1930s by Dr Edward Bach, which can have very soothing effects. There are thirty-eight different flower remedies, each suited to a different state of mind. The flower remedy Hornbeam is used for weariness of mind and body, Gorse for hopelessness, Mustard for depression, Gentian for despondency, Mimulus for fear, Aspen for anxiety, Honeysuckle for living in the past, Impatiens for irritability, and Cherry Plum for the deterioration of the mind. A mixture known as Rescue Remedy can be used for shock or sorrow or bad news. They are not habit-forming and do not interfere with medical treatment.

I have been told that the symptoms suffered when people come off their tablets are a return to the original anxiety. Is this true?

As explained in Chapter 2, the simple answer is no. This fallacy is rapidly losing credence. The withdrawal illness can easily resemble a return to any pre-tablet anxiety state, but the symptoms strike people who have had no previous history of anxiety as well as those who have.

Anxiety coping can help, particularly if it includes that all-important abdominal breathing. But other methods may be less advisable. Anxiety training sometimes involves a relaxation technique in which the muscles are flexed, which is not a good idea during a withdrawal programme. Remember that benzodiazepines are very powerful muscle relaxants, and the body's muscles are tormented enough from the withdrawal without adding to it by systematically flexing every muscle in the body. Avoid this kind of exercise until well after the tablets have been stopped; concentrate instead on more gentle exercise.

Why do some doctors reject the idea of a withdrawal illness caused by coming off these tablets?

In the early 1980s many doctors refused to believe that tablets had made people ill, and even today there are still some who do not comprehend the grim realities of the misery and heartache caused by these tablets. If doctors have been issuing prescriptions year after year you could hardly expect them to announce suddenly that it is their chosen treatment that has been making you feel so ill. If a doctor helps a patient in a genuine and supportive way through tablet withdrawal he or she will have a friend for life – even if he or she has been dishing out the tablets continuously. It could be said that if the problem were fully understood you would not be reading this book!

My mother is seventy-six. Surely she is too old to stop her tablets?

That depends. As people get older they need fewer tablets, so one compromise could be to reduce the level. One of our favourite letters came from the daughters of an eighty-six-year-old pensioner: they and their GP thought that their mother was beginning to suffer from senile dementia, and they were actively considering placing her in a nursing home to finish off her days. Then the daughters realised that their mother was on a benzodiazepine drug, so they slowly helped her to reduce her dose to a very low level. She sprang to life and once more took up her old hobbies of painting and drawing; she has regular tea parties with her pals, and laughs and jokes. Maybe that shows that you are never too old.

What does sadden me is that many of the elderly living in nursing homes are routinely given tablets to induce sleep: 'geriatric junkies', the newspapers have called them. If you have a relative in such an establishment, please keep a careful eye on them to make sure they are not being dosed with tablets.

Since starting on tranquillisers I have become forgetful, though I used to have a responsible job. I cannot imagine ever returning to a job like that.

The tablets do make people forgetful. In a study reported by Professor Malcolm Lader a woman's IQ was measured before and after withdrawal of the tranquilliser. Once off her tablets it jumped by twenty points. So don't give up hope of returning to your job.

What does taking it slowly really mean?

The vital importance of a slow withdrawal programme has been constantly emphasised throughout this book. The time it will take (excluding the time spent in repairing your general health through diet and breathing before you start) will vary between six and eighteen months, depending on the level of stress in your life. Be prepared for this from the start. The alternative is confusion, convulsions and toxic psychosis – a form of drug-induced madness.

Professor Malcolm Lader of the Institute of Psychiatry in London told one conference that he had never known anybody to die when they go cold turkey after taking heroin; but he had known people to die when they abruptly halted their tranquillisers. He also said that he had brought people slowly off some tranquillisers even if they had only taken them for two weeks!

How often should tablets be reduced?

On average people should be able to cut down their tablets every two weeks. Being tablet-free in the shortest possible time should not be the aim. That, sadly, often results in people not only going back on their tablets but remaining on them. But remember that the reduction intervals should depend on the stresses and strains in your life. Some people may wish to reduce once a week, though that would seem to be too quick for the majority. The preferred absolute minimum interval is ten days. Others may want to do it more slowly and cut down every three weeks or even every month. It really depends on the individual and what you are happy with.

How much should you reduce by?

The examples in Chapter 7 will give a clear indication about the level of reduction from a specific daily dose. But as a general rule the reductions should be in stages of no more than one-eighth of the normal daily dose. It can be fiddly having to break small tablets into halves or quarters, but the trouble is well worth it. A lot of people have found their own ingenious ways of coming off tablets, and their tenacity and enterprise must be admired. Some use a nail file to remove fragments of the tablet, while others take a pestle and mortar to grind their tablets into a fine powder and then remove tiny amounts. If you have difficulty doing this, ask the pharmacist – though he or she will probably need a note from your doctor. Likewise a pharmacist can dilute your medication if it is prescribed in liquid form.

Capsules, however, present a further problem. Some people carefully open the gelatine shells, remove some of the powder and take what remains. Although many people have achieved success using that method, the difficulty is that there is no way of knowing whether you are taking the actual drug or just the filler. So removing, for instance, one-quarter of the powder is no guarantee that one-quarter of the drug content is being removed. It is very much a trial and error thing, but I do know that some people would rather persevere and take their chances by doing it this way.

Which plan is for you?

The following four chapters cover withdrawing from a whole range of medication. Chapter 7 deals with the most common tranquilliser of all, Valium or Diazepam. Even if you do not take this particular drug it is worthwhile reading this chapter because later on I shall be discussing a switch to Diazepam as part of a withdrawal package. Chapter 8 describes a plan for withdrawing from Lorazepam or Ativan – a drug which has more problems associated with it than all the other tranquillisers put together. If you take short-acting tablets such as Triazolam or Halcion you will also find this chapter useful. Chapter 9 covers sleeping pills, and other benzodiazepines not already dealt with. Chapter 10 talks about drugs that are not the chief concern of this book, but about which some people may nevertheless welcome a little advice: antidepressants, barbiturates and the major tranquillisers.

Let me reassure you that reducing tablets in the way outlined in this book is completely safe. None of the frightening symptoms mentioned will be experienced if you follow a slow reduction programme.

One last word of advice: don't let concentrating on your own particular withdrawal regime make you lose sight of your breathing exercises and new eating habits. If you let these slip you may have a setback, so give yourself the best possible chance to start with.

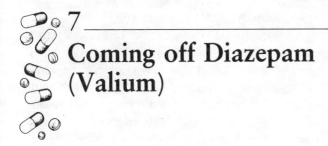

7
Coming off Diazepam (Valium)

First decide whether you are going to reduce fortnightly, every three weeks, or whatever. It all depends on what you think you will feel comfortable with. Remember too that Diazepam comes in many different guises – if you are unsure what your medication really is, look in the list on p. 146.

Most users will be taking between 15mg and 30mg daily, usually in three separate doses – for example, three of either the 5mg or 10mg tablets each day, taken morning, afternoon and evening. There will also be others taking up to 90mg a day, possibly even more in some rare cases. If you take more than the normal daily dose just follow this plan in the same way: everything that has been written about slow withdrawal applies to people on higher doses.

Usually, however, it is possible for them to reduce in larger increments to start off with. If you take over 50mg a day you should be able to cut out 5mg in one go without any trouble. People taking between 30mg and 50mg daily should be able to reduce by 4mg each time. Depending on your daily dose, continue reducing at your chosen intervals at the level of 4mg or 5mg until you reach a daily dose of 30mg.

When you reach 30mg daily, or if you are starting at

that point, reduce for the time being in stages of just 2mg. Hopefully your doctor will co-operate and supply you with a mixture of 2mg and 5mg tablets to enable you to follow an easy regime without difficulty.

Although Diazepam is of course available in 10mg tablets it is better to stick to the two lower-dose tablets to avoid any chance of confusion. Don't forget that two of the 5mg tablets, or for that matter five of the 2mg tablets, contain just as much Diazepam as one of the 10mg tablets. It might look as though you are taking more, but I can assure you that you are not.

If you have been taking, for example, 30mg of Diazepam daily this amount must be taken each day no matter how you feel, because it is important to regulate the amount of drug going into your system: it will help to stabilise your brain. Some people often go for a day or two without taking the full amount because they don't feel too bad. But then they are hit by a real hiccup in their health a few days later and quickly reach for the tablets. So if you have been missing out tablets on odd days, or increasing the daily dose on an ad hoc basis, give yourself a period of time on your normal dose. Spend, for instance, two weeks on a strict daily dose to help prepare your body for the withdrawal programme.

As most people will be taking tablets in three doses a day we will stick to that regime in the examples that follow. But the same general principles apply if you take your tablets twice a day or for that matter four times daily. Just adapt the plan to your own circumstances.

In the examples given the tablets have been withdrawn in the order of afternoon, morning and evening. But you can choose any order of rotation that you feel happy with.

Example 1: 60mg of Diazepam daily, taken as three times 20mg

Day 1:

morning	20mg
afternoon	15mg
evening	20mg

total 55mg daily

If you feel that reducing in 5mg stages is too much for you there is no harm in cutting down at a slower rate, such as 4mg, 3mg or even 2mg stages. It is far better to take it at a rate you feel you can handle.

After your selected reduction period (for example two weeks later):

morning	15mg
afternoon	15mg
evening	20mg

total 50mg daily

The reductions are being rotated, so continue cutting down by 5mg stages until you reach 30mg a day in total. At that stage follow Example 3, which has a starting point of 30mg, because from that point the reductions will be much smaller than the previous 5mg ones.

Example 2: 45mg of Diazepam daily, taken as three times 15mg

Day 1:

morning	15mg
afternoon	11mg
evening	15mg

total 41mg daily

This is a reduction of 4mg, which most people taking over 30mg should be able to tolerate. But again, if it makes you feel ill simply cut down by levels of 2mg or 3mg. Continue to reduce in 4mg stages until you reach:

morning	11mg
afternoon	11mg
evening	11mg
	total 33mg daily

Instead of the next reduction being 4mg it will be more convenient to cut out 3mg. That will bring you nicely to a round total of 30mg and you can then follow Example 3, which is for those starting at 30mg a day.

Example 3: 30mg of Diazepam daily, taken as three times 10mg

Day 1:

morning	10mg
afternoon	8mg
evening	10mg
	total 28mg daily

Remain there for your chosen period and then do the following:

morning	8mg
afternoon	8mg
evening	10mg
	total 26mg daily

Continue to reduce in the same way at the next changeover date:

morning	8mg
afternoon	8mg
evening	8mg
	total 24mg daily

Next:

morning	8mg
afternoon	6mg
evening	8mg
	total 22mg daily

Then:

morning	6mg
afternoon	6mg
evening	8mg
	total 20mg daily

Keep it up – you are doing well:

morning	6mg
afternoon	6mg
evening	6mg
	total 18mg daily

Next:

morning	6mg
afternoon	4mg
evening	6mg
	total 16mg daily

You are now virtually halfway home. Remember to keep up your daily abdominal breathing exercise and the healthy eating.

So far you have been cutting down in stages of 2mg. Now that you have reached 16mg the reductions should be in steps of 1mg. Remember, though, that if 1mg reductions are too much for you to handle there is no harm in cutting down by smaller amounts. This is what you do next:

morning   5mg
afternoon   4mg
evening   6mg
          total 15mg daily

Continue to reduce in the same way by reductions of 1mg each time until you reach a total daily dose of 5mg. At that stage the recommended reduction stages will be in stages of just 0.5 (½) mg. The next example, for people taking a daily dose of 15mg, will give you guidance should you need it. But by now you should have the routine well under control.

Example 4: 15mg of Diazepam daily, taken as three times 5mg

In this example we are continuing with the idea of three equal doses each day. But your own dose could be in two or four divided doses, or even as a single dose at, for instance, bedtime. Take the general idea and adapt it to your own situation.

Those of you continuing the reduction programme from higher dosages should remain at your preferred time intervals. For those just joining the programme, cut down in the following way weekly, fortnightly, monthly or whatever, depending on your own circumstances.

morning	5mg
afternoon	4mg
evening	5mg
	total 14mg daily

Then:

morning	4mg
afternoon	4mg
evening	5mg
	total 13mg daily

Continue:

morning	4mg
afternoon	4mg
evening	4mg
	total 12mg daily

Next:

morning	4mg
afternoon	3mg
evening	4mg
	total 11mg daily

It's going really well! Carry on:

morning	3mg
afternoon	3mg
evening	4mg
	total 10mg daily

Then:

morning	3mg
afternoon	3mg
evening	3mg
total	9mg daily

Continue:

morning	3mg
afternoon	2mg
evening	3mg
total	8mg daily

After that:

morning	2mg
afternoon	2mg
evening	3mg
total	7mg daily

Carry on:

morning	2mg
afternoon	2mg
evening	2mg
total	6mg daily

Then:

morning	2mg
afternoon	1mg
evening	2mg
total	5mg daily

Now that you are down to 5mg of Diazepam daily – after possibly trying in vain many times before to reduce your tablets – it will be obvious that this slow reduction plan has really paid dividends. You should be feeling a lot better, particularly if you have continued to follow the eating plan and the abdominal breathing exercise. But even if you don't feel on top of the world you will not feel anything like as bad as you did when you were on a higher dose of tablets all those months ago. By now your memory should be functioning a lot better and you should be feeling more alert. Please don't worry if you still feel unwell: we are all individuals and we all recover at different rates – *but we do all recover.*

Withdrawal of low doses

At this stage people on prescribed low daily doses of Diazepam can join in. Some people take only 2mg or 3mg a day and have tried to come off even that level, but failed. If that applies to you, please take comfort from the fact that you are not alone. If you have read all this chapter you may be wondering why you are unable to come off what seems to be a small amount compared to those readers who are starting off at a daily dose of 50mg, 60mg or even 90mg. The reason is that your brain becomes tolerant to the drug irrespective of whether you take a small or large dose. I can promise you it has nothing to do with being weak-willed or inadequate. So to those of you on small doses, welcome to our plan and good luck. To those continuing the journey, good luck as you head along the home strait.

From now on the reductions are going to be in stages of 0.5 (½) mg, which involves the tricky job of cutting 2mg tablets into quarters (see p. 99). If you are unable to cut up the tablets ask your doctor about liquid Diazepam.

Example 5: 5mg of Diazepam daily, taken as 2mg morning, 1mg afternoon, 2mg evening

morning	1.5 (1½) mg
afternoon	1 mg
evening	2 mg
	total 4.5 (4½) mg daily

Then:

morning	1.5 (1½) mg
afternoon	1 mg
evening	1.5 (1½) mg
	total 4 mg daily

After that:

morning	1 mg
afternoon	1 mg
evening	1.5 (1½) mg
	total 3.5 (3½) mg daily

Continuing reducing until nothing is left. Congratulations on reaching this point. Many people who have followed this plan have written to tell me that they never believed they could give up their tablets. They had the determination and the willpower – all that was lacking was something to guide them along the way. The final stage is to read Chapter 11, to ensure that you never head this way again.

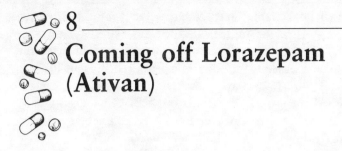

8

Coming off Lorazepam (Ativan)

A problem drug

Experts agree that there are many problems associated with coming off Lorazepam. But in this chapter I am going to describe how it is possible to escape from this drug without experiencing any frightening or severe symptoms.

Lorazepam is often known by its main brand name, Ativan, but there is also a host of other brand names which are all listed on p. 146. Although Lorezepam is a 'minor tranquilliser' that does not in any way mean that it is mild. A lot of people assume that is so, because it comes in seemingly low strengths of 1mg and 2.5 (2½) mg tablets, and they have believed that they are taking nothing more than a gentle, harmless, low-strength relaxant. It is in fact an extremely potent drug, and Dr Heather Ashton has warned that its high potency has not been fully appreciated by many doctors. I have even heard eminent consultants describe Lorazepam as harmless and non-addictive: take their word at your peril.

Its anxiety-relieving activity is estimated to be ten times that of Diazepam. So a person taking what appears to be a small dose of 3mg of Lorazepam each day may actually be taking the equivalent of 30mg of Diazepam. And a person taking three of the 2.5 (2½) mg Lorazepam tablets, which is not at all uncommon, is taking the equivalent of

75mg of Diazepam. That, suggests Dr Ashton, is greatly in excess of the amount needed for most anxiety states.

'I have more trouble bringing people off Lorazepam than all the other tranquillisers put together,' said Professor Malcolm Lader at a conference I attended. More recently Professor Lader said, on a BBC television programme devoted to Lorazepam, 'When somebody comes into my office and says that they have been trying to stop their Lorazepam my heart sinks.' I and most people who have worked in this area of health can confirm that Lorazepam is the real problem drug among long-term tranquilliser users. Most of the disturbing stories which have captured the headlines over the years, or which have been related to me, have involved this drug. There is a real danger that sudden discontinuation of Lorazepam will produce severe withdrawal reactions – some people have even been known to suffer fits.

That information was not meant to scare you, but rather to stress how absolutely essential slow withdrawal is in this context. Even Lorazepam will not give rise to withdrawal symptoms if you follow the Escape Plan faithfully. Once you understand what is happening and why it is happening, it is much easier to do something about it. Dynamite is dangerous stuff in the wrong hands, but handled by an explosives expert it is safe. By fully understanding Lorazepam you can ensure your own safety when you decide to come off it.

Why is Lorazepam different?

Lorazepam was introduced in the 1970s because some of the existing tranquillisers could cause round-the-clock sedation – the drug remained in the body for long periods and left users feeling oversedated. Lorazepam was seen as an answer to this problem because it is a shorter-acting drug and its effects wear off after a few hours. The new drug was regarded as a major breakthrough; at last, it was felt, there was an effective tranquilliser that would not cause hangover effects. During the 1980s it became the second most popular tranquilliser in the UK after Diazepam.

When Lorazepam is used in the correct way – for no more than a few days, or a week at the most – it does indeed avoid the hangover effect. It can therefore be very useful in many situations, particularly for somebody who has a job or a family to look after and needs to remain alert. The problem is that many people become tolerant to the drug within a few weeks of starting a course of treatment. They then suffer from withdrawal symptoms on a day-to-day basis when the effects wear off. A person takes a Lorazepam in the morning, and by late afternoon their body craves another tablet to keep withdrawal symptoms away. In our organisation we generally advise users of Lorazepam to try to space out their daily dose at eight-hourly intervals so that they take some of the tablet three times a day. In this way there will always be some of the drug in the bloodstream, which in turn will help keep the symptoms in check.

Two ways to withdraw from Lorazepam

The first method involves very, very slowly cutting down by literally shaving small fragments off each tablet. This presents difficulties because the tablets are quite small to start with. I will call this the Lorazepam withdrawal method.

The second way is to switch from Lorazepam to a longer-acting medicine, Diazepam, and then gradually withdraw from the new drug. I will call that the substitution method.

Which one do you choose?

That really must depend on you. If you are not feeling too bad and are reasonably satisfied with the quality of your life you may prefer to stick with the tablet that you know so well and slowly withdraw from it. On the other hand, if you are already feeling unwell and have difficulty in coping with life, then a switch to Diazepam is a reasonable way forward. Many thousands of people who were convinced that they would be trapped on Lorazepam for ever have finally succeeded in becoming tablet-free using the substitution method. You will obviously need the support of your doctor for whichever way you feel appropriate in your own case.

Why switch tablets?

Earlier I described the brain's own natural 'tranquilliser reservoir'. What happens with Lorazepam in simple terms is that, because the tablet is shorter-acting, the brain's reservoir is continually at the low-level mark and needs to be regularly topped up. By switching to a longer-acting tablet the reservoir remains at a more stable level and this reduces or eliminates the day-to-day symptoms; certainly there will be no severe symptoms.

Dr Heather Ashton studied thirty-five patients who had each been taking Lorazepam for many years – the average was sixteen years' use. Over three-quarters of the group told her they felt better or did not experience any deterioration in symptoms when they switched tablets. The others experienced some temporary drowsiness or an increase in anxiety, but even these were coped with by adjusting the dosages of Diazepam.

Hopefully you will by now have some idea which route you wish to follow, so let me discuss the two methods in more detail.

Lorazepam withdrawal method

Most people take 2mg or 3mg of Lorazepam daily. With a sharp knife or a nail file you can slice a small amount off one of the tablets. Aim to cut away no more than one-eighth of a tablet. This may seem such an insignificant amount, but that's the whole idea: the point is to trick your brain into not realising that any of the drug has been removed. It might make life easier if you remove one-eighth from a week's supply of tablets in one go, and keep them in a clearly marked container.

If you take three 1mg tablets a day, your first reduction could look something like this:

morning	1 mg
afternoon	0.88 (7/8) mg
evening	1 mg
	total 2.88 (27/8) mg daily

Stay on that level for a period that you feel comfortable with. It might be a week, ten days, two weeks, three weeks or even a month. Reductions every two weeks are the average. Then remove one-eighth from the morning Lorazepam as well. Your new daily dosage would then be:

morning	0.88 (⅞) mg
afternoon	0.88 (⅞) mg
evening	1 mg

total 2.75 (2¾) mg daily

After your selected interval cut the evening tablet as well, so that one-eighth will have been removed from all three, making a daily dosage of 2.63 (2⅝) mg. Don't listen to well-intentioned people who tell you it can be done faster. The reductions you have followed will have been so small that you should not have noticed any difference in the way you feel – but you are already safely on your way off Lorazepam.

The above example was for people taking 3mg of Lorazepam a day. If your daily dosage is higher – 5mg, say, or 7.5 (7½) mg – it is usually possible to start off by reducing in 0.25 (¼) mg stages in the way described above. But when you reach a daily total of 3mg you will be well advised to switch to the smaller reduction stages of just one-eighth.

If you take the 2.5 (2½) mg (yellow) tablets ask the doctor to prescribe an equivalent number of the 1mg (blue) tablets, because it is much better to cut down on those. And ask whether the 0.5 (½) mg tablets are available – that will help even more.

As usual, don't forget your breathing exercises and healthy eating.

Substitution method using Diazepam

Let us say you currently take 3mg a day of Lorazepam, and you feel ill. In fact the days when you feel unwell easily outnumber those when you do not feel too bad. You may even feel ill day after day after day. The chances are, therefore, that you will feel just as bad or worse if you attempt to reduce by even a small amount. So you feel well and truly trapped on your Lorazepam – ill while you take them, but too unwell to stop them.

The reason is that you are already, in all probability, suffering from withdrawal symptoms on a day-to-day basis, so the symptoms can become worse if the dose gets lower. You may want to try to reduce very slowly in the way outlined above, and if necessary put up with any withdrawal symptoms just to get off the tablets. But if you are too ill even to consider coming down off the Lorazepam, we have to think of another safe escape route. The best one devised so far means switching from Lorazepam to Diazepam.

If you use this substitution method it is important to remember that you need to take 10mg of Diazepam for each 1mg of Lorazepam. Some people are initially alarmed by the thought of taking what appears to be a 'high' dose of Diazepam, but careful studies have shown that 10mg is the amount needed to compensate for 1mg of Lorazepam. When this substitution method fails, it is invariably because insuffucient Diazepam has been given. On the other hand, many people who have carefully followed the substitution method are now off their tablets, often for the first time in many years.

Some people have said they are addicted to Lorazepam, and are worried about switching over because they fear becoming addicted to Diazepam. The thing is do not worry about it – the purpose of this whole plan is to allow you to escape for ever from any brain-altering or addictive drugs. Switching over should be seen as a means to an end.

You will need the co-operation of your doctor, so go along to the surgery to discuss your withdrawal plan. Even if the doctor is not fully familiar with withdrawal procedures, he or she can still be a great support by keeping a regular watch on your general health. Having your blood pressure, temperature, pulse and so on taken at regular intervals during the withdrawal programme is very reassuring.

If the doctor agrees to your using the substitution method, ask for a supply of 2mg and 5mg Diazepam tablets. They are different colours, so you will not get them mixed up.

In this example we are switching over from 3mg of Lorazepam to 30mg Diazepam.

Day 1:

morning	1mg	Lorazepam
afternoon	10mg	Diazepam
evening	1mg	Lorazepam

Remain on the above regime for four days, paying attention as always to abdominal breathing and healthy eating.

Day 5:

morning	10mg	Diazepam
afternoon	10mg	Diazepam
evening	1mg	Lorazepam

On day 8 or 9:

morning	10mg	Diazepam
afternoon	10mg	Diazepam
evening	10mg	Diazepam

Your tablet substitution is complete. You should be feeling reasonably well, but if you feel you have gone slightly downhill please do not worry. Once the Diazepam builds up in your system you will feel much better. Most people switch over from Lorazepam to Diazepam with few or no problems and wonder why they did not do it years before. Some people, thankfully a minority, need to switch over a longer period of time. I have even known people who 'played for safe' and took slightly more Diazepam – 33–36mg instead of 30mg – just to see them through those early days. They quickly got rid of the extra once they felt settled.

Remember that you will not suffer from severe withdrawal symptoms if you apply this substitution method correctly. If you do suffer from any symptoms it will help if you concentrate on the abdominal breathing exercise. If you do slip downhill a little, please be patient and allow a week or two for the substitution to work: you will be well rewarded.

The example above referred to people taking 3mg of Lorazepam daily. But it is quite easy to work out an individual programme, no matter what your daily dose. If, for example, you take 0.5 (½) mg of Lorazepam three times daily (total 1.5 (1½) mg), you would switch over in the way described above to end up on 15mg of Diazepam (three of the 5mg tablets).

If you have been taking higher doses of Lorazepam, say between 5mg and 10mg, it is much better to reduce the Lorazepam gradually until 4mg a day or preferably 3mg is reached before switching over. Alternatively, some people prefer to convert 4mg of Lorazepam into 40mg of Diazepam.

When you have been taking your Diazepam for a little time, say two or three weeks, you can then embark on your reduction programme as described in Chapter 7. Remember that the reduction intervals will greatly depend on the stresses and strains of your life and are your decision alone.

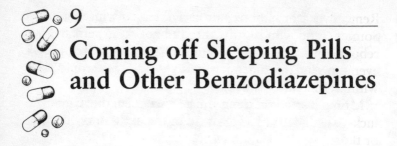

9
Coming off Sleeping Pills and Other Benzodiazepines

So far we have dealt only with the most popular tranquillisers, Diazepam (Valium) and Lorazepam (Ativan). Close relatives of those particular drugs are sleeping pills such as Nitrazepam (Mogadon), Temazepam (Normison, Euphypnos), Triazolam (Halcion) and Flurazepam (Dalmane). They are all from the benzodiazepine family.

Withdrawal from sleeping pills alone

There is a fairly high risk that people attempting to withdraw from sleeping pills will resume their tablets. Why is this? Very often, long-term users of sleeping pills report that they manage to get only a few hours' sleep – three, four or if they are lucky, five hours (in reality, however, people sleep more than they imagine). When they come off their sleeping pills they suffer even worse insomnia, maybe not getting any sleep at all. A typical and understandable reaction is: 'I was getting a few hours' sleep with my tablets – now I am not getting any sleep at all. Therefore I must need the tablets after all.'

The problem is that stopping sleeping pills too quickly causes what is known as rebound insomnia. It is hard to convince people that if they put up with this rebound insomnia for a while their sleep pattern will in time return.

Remember that nobody has ever died from lack of sleep. Some people will, unfortunately, have to experience this rebound insomnia as the price for being tablet-free. But the eventual reward is far more relaxing and refreshing sleep without the aid of drugs.

Michelle took sleeping pills for five years and, if she was lucky, slept for four hours a night – often it was only two or three. When she cut out her sleeping pills she felt really ill and did not sleep at all. Now she sleeps like a log every night and does not need so much as a glass of warm milk as a nightcap. It was the tablets themselves that were keeping her awake more than half the night – but nobody ever told Michelle. Thousands of people have said they sleep better than ever after stopping their sleeping pills. Perhaps if they were called keep-you-awake pills the reality of these hypnotic drugs would dawn on us!

Withdrawal from both tranquillisers and sleeping pills

Although it should not happen, as mentioned earlier many people are prescribed tranquillisers in the daytime as well as sleeping pills for use at bedtime. There are several ways of tackling this situation:

1. Slowly come off the daytime tranquilliser and then tackle withdrawal, again slowly, from the sleeping tablet
2. Slowly come off the sleeping pill, and when that is complete start to withdraw from the tranquilliser. In this regime it is possible to move the evening tranquilliser gradually closer to bedtime, so it helps to act as a sleeping pill

3. Using the chart on p. 124, gradually convert both your daytime tranquilliser and sleeping pill to Diazepam, so that you take just one type of tablet.

You will have to decide which method is best in your own circumstances. It is worth giving the question some thought before embarking on a withdrawal regime – remember, there is no hurry, and patience is usually well rewarded.

Coming off other benzodiazepines

The basic rules about withdrawal, as laid down in Chapter 6, apply to all benzodiazepines. Good diet and proper breathing are also essential elements. The general precept is that no more than one-eighth of a tablet should be withdrawn at any reduction stage. There are, however, a number of problems for people using some of the benzodiazepines. Some are available in a limited range of strengths, some are hard, sugar-coated tablets which are difficult to break into halves or quarters, and many are in capsule form.

Chapter 1 included a list of all benzodiazepines by generic name and indicated the strengths and forms in which they are available (see p. 22). Using that information you should be able to work out whether you can use a mixture of different strengths to apply the withdrawal regime to your own particular medication. Clobazam, for example, is available in just one strength, a 10mg capsule. Quite clearly it is difficult to achieve a gradual tapering off regime using just a single-strength capsule. Chlordiazepoxide, on the other hand, is available in tablet form in strengths of 5mg, 10mg and 25mg, as well as in a 10mg capsule. That does offer scope for a controlled withdrawal programme, using a mixture of different-strength tablets.

These limitations can often be overcome by switching from an existing tranquilliser or sleeping pill to Diazepam, which is more versatile. Chapter 8, dealing with the withdrawal of Lorazepam, gives precise details of how to switch to Diazepam.

There is another good reason why a switch to Diazepam makes a lot of sense. Chapter 8 described how, because Lorazepam is a short-acting drug, it can cause people to suffer withdrawal symptoms on a daily basis. It is not the only short-acting benzodiazepine that gives rise to withdrawal problems – others include Triazolam and Alprazolam. So if your doctor or pharmacist confirms that the particular drug you take is one of the short-acting variety, consider switching to Diazepam. The lists below are a useful starting point.

Long-acting benzodiazepines

- O Clobazam
- O Clorazepate
- O Chlordiazepoxide
- O Diazepam
- O Flunitrazepam
- O Flurazepam
- O Medazepam
- O Nitrazepam
- O Prazepam

Medium/short-acting benzodiazepines

O Alprazolam (very short-acting)
O Bromazepam
O Lorazepam
O Ketazolam
O Loprazolam
O Lormetazepam
O Oxazepam
O Temazepam
O Triazolam (very short-acting)

These are the recommended substitution rates:

Old drug			Diazepam
0.5 (½) mg	Alprazolam	=	10mg
6mg	Bromazepam	=	10mg
25mg	Chlordiazepoxide	=	10mg
20mg	Clobazam	=	10mg
15mg	Clorazepate	=	10mg
1mg	Flunitrazepam	=	10mg
15–30mg	Flurazepam	=	10mg
15–30mg	Ketazolam	=	10mg
1–2mg	Lormetazepam	=	10mg
1–2mg	Loprazolam	=	10mg
10mg	Medazepam	=	10mg
10mg	Nitrazepam	=	10mg
20mg	Oxazepam	=	10mg
10–20mg	Prazepam	=	10mg
20mg	Temazepam	=	10mg
0.5 (½) mg	Triazolam	=	10mg

Triazolam is available in 125mcg (microgram) and 250mcg tablets. This means that two of the 250mcg or four of the 125mcg tablets are each equivalent of 10mg of Diazepam.

Example

If you normally take one of the 250mcg tablets each night, you will need to take as a substitute 5mg of Diazepam. This could be done by starting with 2.5 (2½) mg of Diazepam plus 125mcg Triazolam. By day four or five you could progress to 5mg of Diazepam and no Triazolam. After two to three weeks on Diazepam, start to reduce that drug too by following the withdrawal programme in Chapter 7.

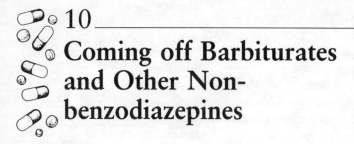

10

Coming off Barbiturates and Other Non-benzodiazepines

Non-benzodiazepines

What about non-benzodiazepine tranquillisers and sleeping pills? These drugs are not really the subject of this book, but since it is estimated that 250,000 people in Britain, mainly the elderly, still take barbiturates, it is only fair to say a few words about them. Here is a list of non-benzodiazepine sleeping pills, relaxants and tranquillisers.

Generic name	Best-known brand names
Barbiturates	Amytal, Soneryl, Tuinal
Buspirone hydrochloride	Buspar
Chloral hydrate	Chloral mixture, Noctec
Chlormethiazole edisylate	Heminevrin
Dichloralphenazone	Welldorm
Meprobamate	Equanil, Meprate
Promethazine hydrochloride	Phenergan
Zopiclone*	Zimovane

*Zopiclone, was introduced on to the UK market in 1990 as a non-benzodiazepine sleeping tablet. The makers claim that there is no evidence of it causing dependence in clinical use. Nevertheless doctors are advised that its use should be for short-term treatment. People taking Zopiclone are also told not to drive or to operate machinery the day after treatment until it has been established that their performance is unimpaired.

Most of the older drugs listed above are now generally unpopular with the medical profession, for reasons explained in Chapter 1. However, some doctors helping people withdraw from benzodiazepine sleeping pills are now using barbiturates in a controlled way. To help the patients deal with rebound insomnia these doctors use a rotation of non-benzodiazepine drugs. A patient may, for instance, be given barbiturates for just one or two nights, then maybe a completely different type of drug for another one or two nights. The idea of this strict rotation is to ensure that the patient does not become hooked on any other medication. It needs strict medical supervision and should not be followed without the help, support and agreement of a medical practitioner.

Antidepressants

Some doctors tend to prescribe antidepressants if patients taking benzodiazepines, or withdrawing from them, complain of feeling depressed. Since depression is one of the possible withdrawal symptoms, this is not entirely surprising. A word of caution here: it is now officially recognised that there can be a withdrawal reaction when antidepressants are stopped.

When an antidepressant is prescribed it takes some time before it begins to work – the full effects may not be felt for six to eight weeks. However, as soon as they are taken you may feel drowsy and experience other effects such as blurred vision and a dry mouth. Unlike benzodiazepines, antidepressants can be dangerous if you overdose. They do not 'cure' depression but mask the symptoms, working on the basis that the depression will eventually lift of its own accord. Because of this, doctors are advised not to prescribe antidepressants for mild depression; unfortunately it would appear that they are given far too readily.

If you do feel depressed you, in consultation with your doctor, must decide whether it is advisable to resort to pills. Many people have said with hindsight that they would have preferred to cope without antidepressants. Some of these drugs have sleep-promoting properties and are given for that reason, but they should not be prescribed merely as a sleeping aid – remember, they are powerful antidepressant drugs, not sleeping pills.

The most common antidepressants

Generic name	Best-known brand names
Amitriptyline	Lentizol, Tryptizol
Clomipramine	Anafranil
Dothiepin	Prothiaden
Doxepin	Sinequan
Fluvoxamine	Faverin
Imipramine	Praminil, Tofranil
Lofepramine	Gamanil
Mianserin	Bolvidon
Trazodone	Molipaxin

Other antidepressants

The first of these is a member of the major tranquilliser group (see below) and it is sometimes prescribed for depression because of its antidepressant properties. Doctors are advised that if it does not produce any response after one week's use it should be withdrawn. The last two are still prescribed, though they are not regarded as the 'drug of choice' by the majority of GPs.

Generic name	Best-known brand names
Flupenthixol	Fluanxol
Phenelzine	Nardil
Tranycypromine	Parnate

Compound drugs

The following are among the compound drugs available – they contain some antidepressant and some tranquilliser. Doctors are advised against prescribing compound medication because it is not possible to adjust the individual components of the tablet.

Compound drugs
Limbitrol
Motipress
Motival
Parstelin
Triptafen

Withdrawing from antidepressant and compound drugs

I have never given a definite yes or no answer to the question of prescribing antidepressants, because it is hard for anybody to comprehend the level of suffering of another individual. If you feel down in the dumps, is it worth resorting to such medication? On the other hand, if you feel suicidal and your life is at risk because of your depression, does it seem inadvisable not to take them? If you follow the advice about abdominal breathing and diet you should hopefully not be faced with the dilemma of deciding.

If you do take benzodiazepines plus antidepressants it is usually better to withdraw first from the tranquilliser or sleeping pill in the way outlined in this book. Then, over a maximum of six to eight weeks, withdraw gradually from the antidepressant.

When people ask for help with withdrawing from the compound medicines they are advised to discuss with their doctor the idea of taking the various compounds separately, so that they can embark on a controlled withdrawal programme. As an example, Limbitrol 5 contains 12.5 (12½) mg of the antidepressant Amitriptyline and 5mg of the tranquilliser Chlordiazepoxide. If you take separate doses of the antidepressant and the tranquilliser you can slowly withdraw from the tranquilliser whilst remaining on the same level of antidepressant. Once off the Chlordiazepoxide you can then look forward to slowly coming off the antidepressant.

Beta blockers

Some doctors have prescribed drugs known as beta blockers to control palpitations and panic attacks during withdrawal. With the controversy surrounding benzodiazepines more of these drugs are now being prescribed not just as part of a withdrawal package but for anxiety too. So what are beta blockers?

Their most common use is in the treatment of angina and high blood pressure and for people who have irregular heart rhythms. It has also been found, however, that beta blockers block the action of a brain chemical noradrenaline – the body's main 'fight or flight' chemical – and so reduce the physical symptoms of anxiety. Although they are not addictive, beta blockers should never be stopped abruptly, as this could cause a heart attack. These drugs must be withdrawn gradually under medical supervision.

When you are offered drugs such as beta blockers and told they are not addictive, you should be made aware just what it is you are taking. How many people would willingly take a form of medication that deliberately affects the working of the heart? In many cases of heart disease and high blood pressure (hypertension) they can be life-saving, but it must also be said that they do not *cure* hypertension. If you have high blood pressure you would be well advised to seek the reasons by looking at your own diet and lifestyle.

Giving beta blockers as an alternative to addictive tranquillisers is a recent trend and time will tell whether it has been worth it. But my own view is that for life problems or anxiety I would not take a drug that slows down such an important organ as my heart.

The most common beta blockers

Generic name	Most common brand names
Propranolol	Inderal LA, Berkolol
Oxprenolol	Trasicor

Major tranquillisers

This group of drugs is beyond the scope of this book, but they are worth a brief mention because they are sometimes given to people experiencing mild anxiety. They are really intended for major psychiatric illnesses such as psychosis or schizophrenia. However, the view among some doctors, particularly some psychiatrists, is that if these drugs can control seriously ill people, milder doses can help with the milder illnesses. Unfortunately they do carry a high risk of side effects, some of which can become permanent. It is not unusual, for instance, for major tranquilliser users to have to take additional drugs just to control the adverse effects. In the psychiatric world they are known as the 'liquid cosh' or 'chemical straitjacket'. They have no doubt helped many people with major mental illnesses to lead something resembling normal lives, but because of the dangers it is questionable whether they have any useful place in the treatment of ordinary everyday life problems.

If you take any of the major tranquillisers listed below you may be wondering whether to come off them. You need to assess the situation carefully, ask your doctor why you are on them and suggest, if it is appropriate, that you would like to come off them. Cut them out over a few weeks – you should not experience withdrawal symptoms from major tranquillisers. If, after a period of weeks, you feel better or no worse, you should not need to resort to them again. But please do not withdraw from these drugs without discussing it with your doctor and asking him or her to monitor your progress. As always, the diet and breathing exercise outlined in Chapters 4 and 5 will greatly help you.

The most commonly prescribed major tranquillisers

Generic name	Best-known brand names
Chlorpromazine	Largactil
Flupenthixol	Depixol
Haloperidol	Fortunan, Haldol, Serenace
Perphenazine	Fentazin
Thioridazine	Melleril
Trifluoperazine	Stelazine

11
Life after Pills

You have just spent some months getting rid of your tablets. The last thing in the world you want is ever to take another one, particularly a powerful brain- or mind-altering drug. Can there ever be a truly safe tranquillising drug? This is very much doubted by a number of leading experts, who feel that such claims should be treated with the utmost caution. The old-fashioned barbiturates were replaced because it was felt that benzodiazepines were safe, but many of you will regret the day you embarked on a course of treatment with them, reassured that at last a 'safe' drug had arrived.

It is hard to imagine that any medicine that dramatically alters the working of the brain can ever be 100 per cent safe. If you are ever offered what is described as a safe and harmless pill, for any illness or condition, just remember what has happened in the past. You need to ask careful questions and try to find information from different sources. A leading consultant psychiatrist once put it this way: '*All* drugs have side effects, and the more powerful the drug the more powerful the side effects.'

The experience of being made ill by prescribed tablets can sometimes make people fearful of taking any medication at all – even everyday painkillers such as aspirin or paracetamol. It is earnestly hoped that you do not become antimedicine altogether because of your past experience.

You will appreciate by now that your illness was caused because the tablets were being used wrongly. That wasn't your fault – you were not given the information needed to allow you to use the tablets in the right way.

There are two questions which people often ask at this stage.

I was off my tablets for six months and then I was suddenly overwhelmed by withdrawal symptoms. Why?

Relapses do happen, which is one of the reasons why the breathing exercises outlined in Chapter 5 need to be practised for many months, along with keeping a careful eye on what you eat and avoiding stressful situations. One possibility is that some of the benzodiazepine may have been deposited in the body's fatty tissue and then suddenly been released. It is also possible that taking the tablets for a long time resulted in changes in the chemistry of the brain which need time to settle down.

Never assume that you will automatically be affected by delayed symptoms, but if you are, try to accept it as a temporary situation. Things do tend to settle down after a few days or a week. Despite the thousands of medical reports and papers written about withdrawal from these tablets, even the academic experts agree there is still a lot to learn.

Now that I am off my tablets I want to know whether I can take them in the future, say in an emergency.

There is a great temptation to give just a blanket no and leave it at that. It would appear that if former long-term users of benzodiazepine again take tablets from that family they very quickly become tolerant to the drug.

This question arose at a conference when it was put to one of the leading experts in pharmacology. The questioner was concerned because she was about to undergo surgery, and benzodiazepine drugs are sometimes used as anaesthetics or as premeds. The reply was that the patient might get away with taking one premed tablet, but nothing more. The best advice in these circumstances – and don't forget this includes dental treatment – is to point out that you have come off benzodiazepine medication and are not eager to be exposed to benzodiazepines in the future (there are usually a whole range of alternatives available to the anaesthetist). It would also make sense to contact a hospital anaesthetist, if relevant, to register your desire to avoid benzodiazepine in the operating theatre.

Avoidance of stress

Earlier in this book I referred to the brain's own 'reservoir' of natural tranquillisers. Now that you are finally off your tablets, you want to ensure that your brain can build up its own 'reservoir' again. This will be greatly helped if you try your best to avoid excessive stress in your life. Just try not to allow things to get you down. Remember: nothing is as important as your own health and wellbeing. Maybe small things around the house or at work would normally have annoyed or angered you. Just say to yourself: forget it, it just isn't worth the worry if it will slow down my complete recovery.

How long complete recovery takes is difficult to say. Certainly, though, the recovery period is controlled by a number of key factors, particularly the breathing exercises and the healthy diet described in Chapters 4 and 5, and staying clear of avoidable stress.

No matter how angry you feel at having been deceived about the true nature of tranquillisers, there is one aspect of stress that you can avoid for yourself. Some years ago I warned in an official report to one of the biggest health authorities in Britain that, if the medical world did not rally around the innocent victims of tranquillisers, the time would come when tablet users sue for damages. That is exactly what did happen: thousands of patients consulted solicitors to seek compensation for their suffering. I have always sounded a cautionary note about medical litigation because at the best of times legal action is stressful – and you are strongly advised to avoid as much stress as possible.

Keeping fit and making friends

Take up gentle exercise, perhaps at a council leisure centre; yoga is ideal, and so are swimming, light aerobics and dancing. The chances are that over the past few years you may have become cut off from family and friends. So any venture into sporting activity will not only help your wellbeing but enable you to meet people.

Make sure that you get enough fresh air, too – dancing may offer welcome social opportunities but it doesn't exactly let you soak up the sunshine! Today many of us spend our days at home or in offices, travelling by car or train and hardly ever seeing the light of day; try to make the effort to get some sunshine – or at least fresh air – on to your skin every day. Dr Damien Downing of York, who has made a detailed study of the part sunlight plays in our health, says it is crucial to our mental and physical wellbeing. In his book *Daylight Robbery* he writes that depression and other mental health problems are much more common in Western society, suggesting that this is partly due to people spending too much time indoors away from the sun. He is not implying that we should spend our time sunbathing, but he does propose that we spend a little time each day out of doors. Sunlight relaxes the muscles, soothes the mind, heals the body and generally helps us to cope with life. Not surprisingly, Dr Downing advises that sunlight should be an essential part of any stress management programme.

Another good way of making friends for those who have become lonely and isolated through their medication is to join an adult education class. Go for enjoyable subjects such as art, pottery, English literature or learning a foreign language, and avoid 'heavy' topics such as psychology or anything that may bring your past health problems flooding back. People have often said that when they come off their tablets they want to join groups to help other victims. Although it is always heartening to observe this genuine desire to help on the part of those who have been through the experience themselves, you may well be better off rejoining the real world and leading an ordinary life.

And don't be tempted to keep telling people, particularly new acquaintances, about your battle with Valium or whatever: not that you should feel anything but proud of your achievement, but because prolonged conversations about health problems can be very boring for others. Remember, too, that when you talk about your struggle with tranquillisers all the memories will come flooding back. Nobody is suggesting that you pretend it didn't happen – but why voluntarily make a big thing about something painful? The goal, after all, is total wellbeing in the future.

Coping with life's problems – without pills

A director of one of the big pharmaceutical companies was once asked about the use of his firm's products and the misery they cause. His reply was quite astonishing and certainly honest: 'If you have a life problem talk it over with a relative, friend, neighbour, counsellor . . . anybody but the doctor. If you go to the doctor, the chances are that he will give you a prescription for one of our products – a tranquilliser.'

He was quite right. In Britain four out of five visits to a GP's surgery end with the writing of a prescription for some kind of medication. That poses a question: should we expect help from doctors when trying to cope with life's problems, great and small? But doctors are busy and overworked; they say they do not have the time to sit and listen to people pour out their problems.

In Oxford, a psychiatrist, Dr José Catalan, headed an interesting research programme involving a group of family doctors. Half the patients were given the usual treatment – medication – and the other half counselling by the GPs themselves. The counselling session conducted by the doctor was to last no more than a few minutes – this was stipulated because the average duration of a GP's consultation in Britain is about six minutes. Dr Catalan established that the people given the short counselling sessions did just as well as those given drugs. (And, of course, the drug group then had to face the task of coming off their tablets.)

If you have a life problem by all means visit the doctor, but do not be surprised if he or she offers a prescription. You cannot always blame the doctor for that – some people feel let down if they come away without a prescription. But try to be aware that there is only a limited number of options that a GP can pursue, particularly if it is an illness caused by stress, anxiety or life problems.

Unfortunately the pharmaceutical company director's solution won't work either. Not so many years ago people shared their problems with friends, relatives, neighbours or the parish priest. Grandparents, parents, brothers and sisters were usually close at hand when that cry for help went out. But with the advent of the nuclear family and the decline in church-going things are very different for many people now, and they have nobody to turn to except the professionals. Look at the amazing 'help' industry that has developed in the USA, with tens of thousands of people having regular sessions with an analyst. Even voluntary counselling agencies are bursting at the seams.

Alternative medicine

So who can you turn to if you want an alternative approach to the treatment offered by your GP? You can choose a doctor who is totally or partly in private practice: he or she may specialise in a particular branch of medicine. There is an army of complementary or alternative doctors and practitioners offering a wide range of treatments. But you must make sure that any practitioner is registered with a recognised professional body. Unfortunately any alternative source of medical help will usually mean paying a fee, though some NHS health areas now have homeopathic units and appointments with those are free. Sadly, few complementary approaches to medicine are provided as part of the NHS in Britain. Many complementary practitioners would like to work within the state system, but it does not happen at the moment, nor is it likely to in the future.

The main sources of alternative or complementary help

are provided by homeopaths, herbalists, acupuncturists and nutritional or ecology doctors. The first appointment is usually the longest (about an hour) and the most expensive; that is because a case history will have to be taken. Follow-up visits are usually much cheaper.

If you do embark on a course of treatment, establish at the start how many visits you are likely to need and the cost. Do not be afraid to point out that you cannot afford treatment indefinitely – that way you will avoid starting treatment and being forced to abandon it part way through the course.

It is impossible to produce a 'league table' of the most successful treatments. You may need to try several approaches – but do persevere, and don't ever consider going back on to pills. Contact the professional bodies to ask for a list of members or practitioners in your area. You can even ask at local health stores whether there are popular or respected practitioners close by.

Sleep – nature's great restorer

Sound healthy sleep is good for us all – an excellent way to relax and deal with stress. But how do you make sure you get it, especially if you have had sleeping problems in the past, and have chosen to withdraw from your pills? First, how much sleep do you need to survive – five hours, seven hours, the usual eight hours, or more? The remarkable thing is that nobody has ever died from lack of sleep. When a certain Hungarian soldier was shot in the head during World War I he completely lost the ability to sleep. Doctors tried all kinds of therapy, from hypnosis to old-fashioned sedatives, but nothing worked. In fact they could not even make him feel drowsy. They predicted that he would not live for long, but the soldier confounded them all. Not only did he complete a full working life, but he lasted well into his retirement in the best of health.

One of the world's leading authorities on sleep, Professor Ian Oswald of Edinburgh University, has said that a few nights' broken sleep, though unpleasant, are not going to have any serious consequences. 'Worrying about not sleeping,' he says, 'is one of the reasons why people stay awake . . . the vicious circle has to be broken.'

Why do we sleep? It is simply a means of recharging our 'batteries' – body tissues are replaced when we slumber. So although sleep is not absolutely essential for survival, it is necessary as a means of restoring our bodies for the next day of activity. Professor Oswald tells of people complaining that they are not fully restored by sleep: in fact, they feel less vigorous during the day. The interesting thing is that studies have shown that those people often sleep just as long as those who are fully refreshed by sleep. One possibility, he says, is that people who feel they have slept poorly may indeed have had less of the particular kind of sleep that restores the body.

In his book *Get a Better Night's Sleep*, written with his wife, Dr Kirstrine Adam, Professor Oswald says the lesson to be learnt is that when we are short of sleep nature takes care of our interests. If we really need sleep and are given the opportunity to do so, then we can rely on nature to give us rest. While lack of sleep may give rise to some unpleasant consequences such as irritability, it is clear that it will not cause any long-term mental or physical ill effects. Interestingly, to look at the other side of the coin, Professor Oswald and Dr Adam revealed that research in the USA has shown that sleeping longer than usual can also lead to inefficiencies and irritability.

Sleep problems, it must be said, are more likely to occur

when there are problems in our lives: redundancy, marriage difficulties, a death in the family, worry about hospital treatment. Such difficulties apart, how can we do the best for ourselves without resorting to the pill bottle?

Simple ways of helping to improve your sleep

Invest in a new bed.   Many people never change their bed until their existing one falls apart. Given that the average person spends a third of his or her life in bed, it is well worth investing in a decent one with a good-quality mattress that will support your body properly and prevent you waking up full of aches and pains.

Try to establish a pattern of going to bed each night at about the same time and getting up each morning at the same time. Routine is a good relaxer.

Make sure your bedroom is at the right temperature for you. Fresh air from an open window is good, provided it doesn't make the room too cold.

Caffeine is one of sleep's greatest enemies. Avoid tea, coffee, cola or any other drinks containing caffeine after about 6pm, since caffeine hangs around in the body for several hours.

Try to avoid late-night thrillers on the television and settle for a sober, sensible book instead to help wind down before slumber.

A glass of warm milk before bedtime is a good nightcap. Use Horlicks if you wish, but I would not recommend drinking chocolate, because it contains caffeine. A small snack at suppertime may also help (see p. 73).

Many people will find doing the breathing exercise described in Chapter 5 for a few minutes will help pave the way for a good sleep.

Alcohol is definitely not a good nightcap, and is in fact

one of the main causes of 'bad sleep'. It will send you to sleep more quickly, but it does cause night-time disturbance.

Daily exercise such as walking, gardening or swimming will help prepare your body for restful sleep.

Many health stores and pharmacies sell a range of non-addictive herbal products which claim to aid sleep. Valerian and passiflora tablets, two of the most popular, are completely safe and well worth trying. Other herbal relaxants are detailed in books specialising in herbal medicine and treatment. (See further reading list.)

A number of herbal teas also help people relax and act as an aid to sleep; the best-known are camomile and lemon balm. Herbal tea can be used in the evenings as an alternative to ordinary tea or coffee. Also available are a number of over-the-counter homeopathic preparations and the famous Bach Flower Remedies.

Do they work? Like most things, they work wonders for some and not at all for others. The thing to do is try them – even if they do no good they will certainly do no harm. Most people should eventually find suitable remedies among the wide range available.

A cautionary note: herbal or homeopathic sleeping or relaxant remedies are not substitutes for prescribed benzodiazepine sleeping pills or tranquillisers. Some people assume, quite wrongly, that it is possible to switch directly from a benzodiazepine to a herbal sleeping remedy. Never attempt this. Even if you take herbal or homeopathic preparations you must continue to follow the slow withdrawal regime outlined in this book or you may suffer acute withdrawal symptoms.

Finally, if nothing works, rather than lie frustrated and angry in bed through lack of sleep it is sometimes better to get up and do something pleasant or useful. That should help take the element of stress out of your sleeplessness.

Looking at a healthy future

People who have taken tablets have been called inad-equates, neurotics, psychotics, depressives, drug addicts, abusers, weak-willed – you name it, the labels have been hurled at them. The truth is, though, that people who have battled their way off their tablets are among the bravest people imaginable. They deserve medals, not insults. Coming off tablets is for many people one of the cruellest illnesses. They have to cope not only with the difficulty of handling the withdrawal symptoms, but also with the disbelief and hostility of those around them – husbands, wives, sons, daughters, brothers, sisters, doctors, nurses, friends, workmates.

This book has been written in the knowledge that those around you will not believe you or even attempt to understand. Of course, if you have had help, so much the better, but regard it as a bonus. As you recover and come alive again those around you will be stunned by your recovery, by the new you. It is so easy to feel bitter and angry, and so understandable. You will know that a bit of help would have spared you the isolation, the lonely, tearful days and nights.

But remember what your goal is – to kick the tablets into touch and to get on with a happy, ordinary life. Use your 'wasted' years as a springboard and learn from your new wisdom. You have worked hard and done well to come off your tablets. Now is the time to think of today and tomorrow – not yesterday. Thank you for reading my Escape Plan – I will be thinking of you all out there.

Appendix: _____
List of Benzodiazepines

Before embarking on the withdrawal of any medication you need to be certain what kind of drug you are taking. The following list gives in alphabetical order both the chemical (generic) and brand names of tranquillisers and sleeping pills available in Australia, the British Isles, Canada, New Zealand, South Africa, and the USA. If the medication you are using is included in this list it is a benzodiazepine.

These lists were accurate at the time of going to press in early 1990, but as new brand names are added they are constantly changing. If your own medication is not listed here, check with a doctor or pharmacist to establish whether or not it is a benzodiazepine.

Brand name	Generic name	Available in
A-poxide	Chlordiazepoxide	USA
Alepam	Oxazepam	AUS
Almazine	Lorazepam	UK
Alodorm	Nitrazepam	AUS
Alupram	Diazepam	UK
Antenex	Diazepam	AUS
Anxon	Ketazolam	UK
Apo Chlordiazepoxide	Chlordiazepoxide	CAN
Apo Diazepam	Diazepam	CAN

Brand name	Generic name	Available in
Apo Flurazepam	Flurazepam	CAN
Apo Lorazepam	Lorazepam	CAN
Apo Oxazepam	Oxazepam	CAN
Arem	Nitrazepam	SA
Atensine	Diazepam	UK
Ativan	Lorazepam	AUS,CAN,NZ,SA,UK, USA
Benzopin	Diazepam	SA
Benzotran	Oxazepam	AUS,NZ
Betapam	Diazepam	SA
Brozam	Bromezepam	SA
Centrax	Prazepam	USA
Cloraze capsules	Clorazepate dip.	USA
Cloraze tablets	Clorazepate dip.	USA
Dalmadorm	Flurazepam	SA
Dalmane	Flurazepam	AUS,CAN,UK,USA
Demetrin	Prazepam	SA
Diaquel	Diazepam	SA
Diatran	Diazepam	SA
Diazemuls	Diazepam	AUS,CAN,NZ,UK
D-Pam	Diazepam	NZ
Dizam	Diazepam	SA
Doral	Quazepam	USA
Dormicum	Midazolam	SA
Dormonoct	Loprazolam	NZ,UK
Doval	Diazepam	SA
Ducene	Diazepam	AUS
E-Pam	Diazepam	CAN
Ethipam	Diazepam	SA
Euhypnos	Temazepam	AUS,NZ,SA
Evacalm	Diazepam	UK
Frisium	Clobazam	AUS,NZ,UK
Halcion	Triazolam	CAN,NZ,SA,UK,USA
Hypnodorm	Flunitrazepam	AUS
Hypnovel	Midazolam	AUS,NZ
Insoma	Nitrazepam	AUS,NZ
Karmoplex	Chlordiazepoxide	SA
Levanxol	Temazepam	SA

Brand name	Generic name	Available in
Lexotan	Bromazepam	AUS,NZ,SA,UK
Librax	Chlordiazepoxide and Clinidium brom.	AUS
Libritabs	Chlordiazepoxide	USA
Librium	Chlordiazepoxide	AUS,CAN,SA,UK, USA
Loftran	Ketazolam	CAN
Loramet	Lormetazepam	SA
Lorapam	Lorazepam	NZ
Lormetazepam	Lormetazepam	UK
Lorzem	Lorazepam	NZ
Lyladorm	Nitrazepam	SA
Mediazepam	Diazepam	SA
Medilium	Chlordiazepoxide	CAN
Meval	Diazepam	CAN
Mitran	Chlordiazepoxide	USA
Mogadon	Nitrazepam	AUS,CAN,NZ,SA,UK
Murcil	Chlordiazepoxide	USA
Murelax	Oxazepam	AUS
Nitrados	Nitrazepam	NZ,UK
Nobrium	Medazepam	UK
Noctesed	Nitrazepam	UK
Noctamid	Lormetazepam	NZ,SA
Normison	Temazepam	AUS,NZ,SA,UK
Notense	Diazepam	SA
Nova Pam	Chlordiazepoxide	NZ
Novoclopate	Clorazepam	CAN
Novodipam	Diazepam	CAN
Novoflupam	Flurazepam	CAN
Novolorazem	Lorazepam	CAN
Novopoxide	Chlordiazepoxide	CAN
Novo-Xapam	Oxazepam	CAN
Ormodon	Nitrazepam	SA
Oxaline	Oxazepam	SA
Oxanid	Oxazepam	UK
Oxpam	Oxazepam	CAN
Ox-Pam	Oxazepam	NZ

Brand name	Generic name	Available in
Pax	Diazepam	SA
Paxadorm	Nitrazepam	SA
Paxane	Flurazepam	UK
Paxipam	Halazepam	USA
PMS Flurazepam	Flurazepam	CAN
PMS Lorazepam	Lorazepam	CAN
PMS Oxazepam	Oxazepam	CAN
Pro-pam	Diazepam	AUS,NZ
Proxam	Oxazepam	SA
Purata	Oxazepam	SA
Reposans 10	Chlordiazepoxide	USA
Restoril	Temazepam	CAN,USA
Rohypnol	Flunitrazepam	AUS,NZ,SA,UK
Scriptopam	Diazepam	SA
Serax	Oxazepam	CAN,USA
Serepax	Oxazepam	AUS,NZ,SA
Serepax Forte	Oxazepam	SA
Solatran	Ketazolam	SA
Solis	Diazepam	UK
Solium	Chlordiazepoxide	CAN
Somnipar	Nitrazepam	SA
Somnite	Nitrazepam	UK
Somnol	Flurazepam Monohydrochlor	CAN
Surem	Nitrazepam	UK
Temodal	Quazepam	SA
Tenax	Chlordiazepoxide	USA
Tensium	Diazepam	UK
Tran-Qil	Lorazepam	SA
Tranqipam	Lorazepam	SA
Tranxene	Clorazepate dip.	AUS,CAN,SA,UK,USA
T-Tab	Clorazepate dip.	USA
Unisomnia	Nitrazepam	UK
Urbanol	Clobazam	SA
Valium	Diazepam	AUS,CAN,NZ,SA,UK, USA
Valrelease	Diazepam	SA,USA

Brand name	Generic name	Available in
Verstram	Prazepam	USA
Vivol	Diazepam	CAN
Xanax	Alprazolam	AUS,CAN,NZ,UK,USA
Xanor	Alprazolam	SA
Zapex	Oxazepam	CAN
Zetran	Chlordiazepoxide	USA

Further Reading List

Tranquillisers/Benzodiazepines

Coming off Tranquillisers and Sleeping Pills, Shirley Trickett SRN, Thorsons, 1986
Women and Tranquillisers, Celia Haddon, Sheldon Press, 1984

General/Nutritional Health

Raw Energy, Leslie and Susannah Kenton, Arrow, 1984
The Wright Diet, Celia Wright, Grafton, 1989
Daylight Robbery, Dr Damien Downing, Arrow, 1988
The Good Health Handbook, Dr Peter Mansfield, Grafton, 1988
Coping with Anxiety and Depression, Shirley Trickett, Sheldon Press, 1989
The British Medical Association Guide to Medicines and Drugs, Dorling Kindersley, 1988
Food Combining for Health, Doris Grant and Jean Joice, Thorsons, 1984

Recommended Academic Reading List

'Benzodiazepine withdrawal: an unfinished story', Dr C H

Ashton MA,DM,FRCP, *British Medical Journal*, 14 April 1984

'Benzodiazepine dependence and withdrawal update', *Drug Newsletter*, No. 31, Wolfson Unit of Clinical Pharmacology, April 1985

'Benzodiazepines in general practice: time for a decision', José Catalan and Dennis H Gath, *British Medical Journal*, 11 May 1985

'Clinical management of benzodiazepine dependence', Anna C Higgitt, Professor M H Lader and P Fonagy, *British Medical Journal*, 14 September 1985

'Anything for a quiet life?', Dr C H Ashton, *New Scientist*, 6 May 1989

'Some problems with benzodiazepines', *Drug and Theraapeutics Bulletin*, Consumers' Association, 25 March 1985

'Lorazepam: a benzodiazepine to choose or avoid?' *Drug and Therapeutics Bulletin*, Consumers' Association, 12 August 1985

'Management of depression in general practice', Professor Sydney Brandon, *British Medical Journal*, 1 February 1986

'Adverse effects of prolonged benzodiazepine use', Dr C H Ashton, Dr D M Davies, Shotley Bridge General Hospital, *Adverse Drug Reaction Bulletin*, No. 118, June 1986

'Dependence on tranquillisers', Professor Malcolm Lader, *Druglink*, May/June 1987

'Hyperventilation and anxiety state', Dr L C Lum, *Journal of the Royal Society of Medicine*, January 1981

'Chronic hyperventilation and its treatment by physiotherapy: discussion paper', R A Cluff MCSP, SRP, *Journal of the Royal Society of Medicine*, October 1984

Useful Addresses

Please enclose an SAE when writing to any of the
organisations listed.

Tranxline
PO Box 20
Liverpool L17 6DS

Tranx UK
25a Masons Avenue
Wealdstone
Middlesex HA3 5AP

Bach Flower Remedies
Mount Vernon
Sotwell
Wallingford
Oxon OX10 0PZ

British Herbal Medicine
    Association
Lane House
Cowling
Keighley
West Yorkshire BB22 0LX

Council for
    Complementary and
    Alternative Medicine
Suite 1
19a Cavendish Square
London W1M 9AD

National Institute of
    Medical Herbalists
41 Hatherley Road
Winchester
Hampshire SO22 6RR

Natural Medicine Society
Edith Lewis House
Back Lane
Ilkeston
Derbyshire DE7 8ET

Society of Homeopaths
2 Artizan Road
Northampton NN1 4HU

Chartered Society of
  Physiotherapy
14 Bedford Row
London WC1R 4ED

Help For Self-Help Groups

A starter-pack is available for professional and lay help groups or agencies. It contains booklets, draft fact-sheets, draft press releases, information data on withdrawal and drugs lists. It also gives many useful tips on starting and effectively running help groups. Compiled by Susan Hill, Information Officer, Tranxline, Liverpool, it is available for £24 if you send a cheque or postal order made payable and forwarded to Tranxline, PO Box 20, Liverpool L17 6DS (Overseas, European, inc. Eire, orders welcome. Cost £28)

Index

abdominal breathing, 57, 58, 87–9
accidents, 40
acidity, 67–8
acupuncture, 141
Adam, Dr Kirstrine, 142
addiction, 50–1
adult education, 138
advertising, 33–5
aggression, side effect, 40
agoraphobia, 51
alcohol, 40, 71, 144
alkaline balance, 67–9
Alprazolam, 22, 123, 124
alternative medicine, 140–1
Amitriptyline, 128, 130
Amytal, 126
anaesthetics, 136
Anafranil, 128
antidepressants, 51, 85, 95
    withdrawing from, 127–30
anxiety: hyperventilation and, 85–6
    relaxation techniques and, 96
    tranquilliser use for, 18, 19, 35, 43
    as withdrawal symptom, 45, 96
Anxon, 23–4
Ashton, Dr Heather, 28, 35, 38, 46–
    7, 58, 111–12, 114–15
aspirin, 134
Ativan, 14, 19
    advertising, 33
    dosage, 24
    withdrawing from, 57, 111–19
    see also Lorazepam
Aztecs, 28

babies, addiction, 48–50
baby battering, 42
Bach, Dr Edward, 95
Bach Flower Remedies, 95, 144
bananas, 72
barbiturates, 29, 47, 134

    withdrawing from, 126–7
BBC, 14, 37–8, 74, 112
beans, 71
beans with cauliflower, 78
beef: hot and cold casserole, 76
beetroot, 68, 72
benzodiazepines, see sleeping pills;
    tranquillisers
benzophenones, 30
bereavement, 35–6
Berkolol, 131
beta-blockers, 95
    withdrawing from, 130–1
Betty Ford Center, 32
blood sugar levels, 73, 80
Bolvidon, 128
brain: addiction to tranquillisers, 26–7
    how benzodiazepines work, 25–6
    Lorazepam and, 114
    recovery from tranquillisers, 136
Brandon, Sydney, 85
breakfast, 73
breastfeeding, 49
breathing: breathing exercises, 57,
    58, 81, 86–8, 135, 143
    hyperventilation, 58, 81–6
    physiotherapy, 88–9
British Journal of Addiction, 12
British Medical Association (BMA),
    14, 37
British Medical Journal, 41–2
The British National Formulary, 18,
    19, 20, 21, 35, 49
Bromazepam, 22, 124
bromides, 29
Buspar, 126
Buspirone hydrochloride, 126
cabbage, 71
caffeine, 70, 143
capsules, reducing, 99
carrots, 72

Carruthers, Dr Malcolm, 65
casserole, hot and cold, 76
Catalan, Dr José, 139
cauliflower, beans with, 78
celery, 72
Central America, 28
cheese, 68
children, tranquilliser prescriptions, 35
chloral, 29
Chloral hydrate, 126
Chloral mixture, 126
Chlorazepate dipotassium, 23
Chlordiazepoxide: in compound medicines, 130
  dosage, 23
  withdrawing from, 122–3, 124
Chlormethiazole edisylate, 126
Chlorpromazine, 133
Clobazam, 23, 122, 123, 124
Clomipramine, 128
Clorazepate, 123, 124
Cluff, Rosemary, 82, 83, 86
coffee, 70, 143
Committee on the Review of Medicines (CRM), 42–3, 44, 45, 47–8.
Committee on the Safety of Medicines (CSM), 18–19, 44
complementary medicine, 140–1
compound drugs, 129–30
Consumers' Association, 19
counselling, 139–40
cucumber, 71
Currie, Edwina, 13

Daily Mail, 30, 31
Daily Mirror, 30
Dalmane, 24, 37, 120
Davies, Stephen, 66–7
delayed symptoms, 135
Depixol, 133
depression, 85, 127–8, 129, 138
Diazepam: dosage, 21, 22
  introduction of, 31
  withdrawal from, 48, 55, 101–10

and withdrawal from Lorazepam, 114–15, 116–19
and withdrawal from other benzodiazepines, 123, 124–5
Dichloralphenazone, 126
diet, 57, 58, 63–80
  alkaline balance, 67–9
  healthy diet, 69–74
  raw food, 65–9
  recipes, 74–80
doctors: alternative medicine, 140–1
  counselling, 139
  ignorance of nutrition, 64
  over-prescribing, 35–7, 139–40
  promotion of benzodiazepines to, 33–5
  reasons for prescribing tranquillisers, 38–9
  sources of drug information, 18, 19
  withdrawal regimes, 91–3, 96–7, 117–18
Dormonoct, 25
dosages, 21–5
  reduction in, 98–9
Dothiepin, 128
Downing, Dr Damien, 137–8
Doxepin, 128
Doyle, Christine, 43–4
drinks, 40, 70, 71, 144
driving, effects of benzodiazepines, 40
Drug and Therapeutics Bulletin, 19
drug companies, 28, 29, 33–4
drug dependency units, 53–5

eggs, 68
Egypt, 28
elderly patients, 21, 97
emergency snack, 80
epilepsy, 18, 48
Equanil, 126
Euphypnos, 120
exercise, 137, 144
  breathing exercises, 57, 58, 81, 86–8, 135, 143

Faverin, 128
Federal Drugs Administration (USA), 43
Fentazin, 133
fish, 68, 71, 73
flower remedies, 95, 144
Fluanxol, 129
Flunitrazepam, 123, 124
Flupenthixol, 129, 133
Flurazepam, 24, 37, 120, 123, 124
Fluvoxamine, 128
Ford, Betty, 32
Foresight, 49
forgetfulness, 40, 97–8
Fortunan, 133
Freud, Sigmund, 32
friendships, 137, 138
Frisium, 23
fruit, 66, 68, 71
fruit salad, 79

Gamanil, 128
Garland, Judy, 32
Gordon, Barbara, 42
grapes, 71
group therapy, 56

Halcion, 25, 120
Haldol, 133
Haloperidol, 133
ham: simple pea and ham soup, 77–8
Hansard, 44
haricot beans: beans with cauliflower, 78
hashish, 28
heart disease, 130–1
Heminevrin, 126
heptodiazines, 30
herbal medicines, 28–9
herbal tea, 71, 144
herbalism, 141, 144
heroin, 53, 98
Herxheimer, Dr Andrew, 19
Hillsborough disaster, 36
Hippocrates, 63, 64
history, 28–31

homeopathy, 140, 141, 144
hospital treatment, 53–5
hot and cold casserole, 76
House of Commons, 44
hyperventilation, 58, 81–6
hypnotics, 18

iatrogenic illness, 51
Imipramine, 128
Inderal LA, 131
insomnia, 18, 19
    prescribing guidelines, 20–1, 43
    side effects of benzodiazepines, 39
    tranquillisers and, 20
    withdrawal from sleeping pills, 120–1, 127
    as withdrawal symptom, 45, 47
    see also sleep
Institute for the Study of Drug Dependence, 34
International Journal of Addiction, 33
iron, 71

Johnson, Colin, 35
Journal of the Royal Society of Medicine, 82

Kenton, Leslie and Susannah, 65–6, 67
Ketazolam, 23–4, 124
Kilroy Silk, Robert, 52–3
Kinross-Wright, Dr John, 30–1

Lacey, Ron, 38, 53, 54–5
lactucin, 71
Larder, Professor Malcolm, 42, 94, 97–8, 112
lamb: hot and cold casserole, 76
Largactil, 133
legal action, 137
lentils: hot and cold casserole, 76
Lentizol, 128
lettuce, 71
Lexotan, 22
Librium: advertising, 34
    dosage, 23

introduction of, 30–1
see also Chlordiazepoxide
Limbritol, 129, 130
litigation, 137
Liverpool, 36
Lofepramine, 128
long-acting benzodiazepines, 47, 123
Loprazolam, 25, 124
Lorazepam, 19, 36
   advertising. 33
   dosage, 21, 24
   introduction of, 112–13
   as a sleeping pill, 20
   withdrawal from, 57, 92, 111–19,
     124
Lormetazepam, 25, 124
Lum, Dr Claud, 83, 84, 85–6

McCartney, Paul, 11
McLeave, Hugh, 30
magnesium, 66–7, 72
major tranquillisers, 131–3
mangoes, 72
Mansfield, Dr Peter, 64
meat, 68, 71, 73
Medazepam, 24, 123, 124
Melleril, 133
Melville, Dr Arabella, 35
memory loss, 40, 97–8
Meprate, 126
Meprobamate, 29, 126
Mianserin, 128
MIND, 37–8, 53
mineral supplements, 74
Minnelli, Liza, 32
Mogadon, 25, 120
Molipaxin, 128
Motipress, 129
Motival, 129
multiple sclerosis, 46
muscles: relaxants, 18, 82, 96
   relaxation exercises, 96

Nardil, 129
National Institute on Drug Abuse
     (USA), 43

National Institute for Mental Health
     (USA), 47
Nellis, Muriel, 32–4
nervous system: how benzodiazepines
     work, 25–6
   raw food and, 66
New England Journal of Medicine,
     48
New Society, 33
Newcastle University, 49, 57–8
News Chronicle, 31
Nitrazepam, 25, 47, 120, 123, 124
Nobrium, 24
Noctec, 126
noradrenaline, 130–1
Normison, 25, 35, 120
nutrition *see* diet
nutrition therapy, 141
nuts, yoghurt with, 80

oatcakes, 78–9
oats, 72
Observer, 43–4
onion soup, 77
Oriental medicine, 65
Oswald, Professor Ian, 142
Oxanid, 24
Oxazepam, 24, 34, 124
Oxprenolol, 131

pain, 84
painkillers, 95, 134
palpitations, 45, 81, 82, 130
panic attacks, 39, 45, 81, 82, 130
Papworth Breathing Exercise, 86–7
Papworth Hospital, 57, 83, 86
paracetamol, 134
Parnate, 129
Parstelin, 129
peas: hot and cold casserole, 76
   simple pea and ham soup, 77–8
pecan nuts, 72
Perphenazine, 133
Perry, Lyn, 34
pharmaceutical industry, 28, 29, 33–
     4
pharmacists, 98–9

Phenelzine, 129
Phenergan, 126
physiotherapy, 88
Porpora, Dr Douglas, 33
porridge, 72
potassium, 71, 72
Praminil, 128
Prazepam, 123, 124
pregnancy, 48–50
prescriptions: guidelines, 18–21
  over-prescribing, 35–7, 139–40
  repeat prescriptions, 36, 43, 50
processed foods, 70
Promethazine hydrochloride, 126
propranolol, 131
Prothiaden, 128
psychiatric wards, 53
psychiatrists, 51, 65, 132
psychoanalysis, 65
Psychopharmacology Bulletin, 47
pyridoxine, 72

Rantzen, Esther, 37, 38
raw food, 65–9, 73
Rawlins, Professor Michael, 41–2,
  57–8
rebound insomnia, 120–1, 127
recipes, 74–80
reduction of tablets, 98–9
Reid, Daniel, 65
relaxants, muscle, 18, 82, 96
relaxation, 87, 96
repeat prescriptions, 36, 43, 50
Roche, 30
Rolling Stones, 12

salads: fruit salad, 79
  green vegetable salad, 75
  raw vegetable salad, 74–5
sedatives *see* sleeping pills;
  tranquillisers
self-help groups, 56
Serax, 34
Serenace, 133
shellfish, 68
shoplifting, 40

short-acting benzodiazepines, 47–8,
  123, 124
side effects, 39–42, 45, 51
Sinequan, 128
sleep, 141–4
  purpose of, 142
  ways of improving, 143–4
  withdrawal from sleeping pills,
    120–1, 127
  see also insomnia
sleeping pills: dosages, 24–5
  effectiveness in long-term use, 43
  how they work, 25–6
  numbers addicted to, 12
  prescribing guidelines, 20–1
  promotion of, 33–5
  uses, 18
  who takes them, 32–3
  withdrawing from, 47, 120–2
Smith, Dr Andrew, 42
snacks, 73, 80, 143
snakeroot, 28–9
Soneryl, 126
soups: onion, 77
  simple pea and ham, 77–8
sports, 137
sprouted seeds and beans, 73
Stelazine, 133
Stewart, Dr Alan, 66–7
stress, 26, 27, 29, 68, 82, 136–7
substitution method: withdrawal
    from Lorazepam, 114–15, 116–
    19
  withdrawal from other
    benzodiazepines, 124–5
suicide, 29, 129
sunflower seeds, 71–2
sunlight, 137–8
symptoms: delayed, 135
  side effects, 39–42, 45, 51
withdrawal, 40–4, 45–9, 51, 93–7,
  135

tablets, reducing, 98–9
Taylor, Elizabeth, 32
tea, 70, 143

herbal, 71, 144
Temazepam, 17
  dosage, 25
  as a tranquilliser, 20
  withdrawing from, 120, 124
That's Life!, 37–8, 53
Thioridazine, 133
Tofranil, 128
tranquillisers: addiction to, 26–7,
    50–1
  dosages, 21–4
  effectiveness in long-term use, 19,
    43
  history, 29–31
  hospital treatment, 53–5
  how they work, 25–6
  lack of public information, 36, 37–
    8
  numbers of users, 12, 38, 42
  over-prescription of, 35–7
  in pregnancy, 48–50
  prescribing guidelines, 18–19
  promotion of, 33–5
  reasons for prescribing, 38–9
  self-help groups, 56
  side effects, 39–42, 45, 51
  uses, 18
  who takes them, 32–3
  withdrawal from sleeping pills and,
    121–2
  withdrawal programme, 90–100
  withdrawal symptoms, 40–4, 45–
    9, 51
  see also individual drugs
Tranxene, 23
Tranxline, 13
Tranycypromine, 129
Trasicor, 131
Trazodone, 128
Triazolam, 25, 120, 123, 124–5
Trifluoperazine, 133
Triptafen, 129
Tryptizol, 128
tryptophan, 72
Tuinal, 126
turkey, 72

Valium, 17, 32
  addiction to, 44
  advertising, 34
  dosage, 22
  introduction of, 31
  side effects, 40–1, 42
  withdrawing from, 101–10
  see also Diazepam
vegetables, 66, 67, 68, 71, 73
  green vegetable sald, 75
  raw vegetable salad, 74–5
vitamin B complex, 71
vitamin B6, 72
vitamin C, 71, 74
vitamin E, 71, 72
vitamin supplements, 74

Watson, Dr George, 65
Welldorm, 126
wheatgerm oil, 72
White House Office of Drug Policy, 43
wholegrains, 71
withdrawal programme:
  antidepressants, 127–30
  beta-blockers, 130–1
  breathing exercises, 57, 58, 81,
    86–8, 135, 143
  Diazepam (Valium), 101–10
  diet, 63–80
  essential ground rules, 90–100
  Lorazepam (Ativan), 111–19
  non-benzodiazepines, 126–7
  other benzodiazepines, 122–5
  sleeping pills, 120–2, 127
withdrawal symptoms, 40–4, 45–9,
    51, 93–7, 135
women and tranquillisers, 32–4
Woodward, Shaun, 38
Wright, Celia, 68–9, 74

Xanax, 22

yoga, 57, 137
yoghurt with nuts, 80

Zimovane, 126
Zopiclone, 126